SYNDEMIC SUFFERING

Advances in Critical Medical Anthropology
Series Editors: Merrill Singer and Pamela Erickson

This book series advances our understanding of the complex and rapidly changing landscape of health, disease, and treatment around the world with original and innovative books in the spirit of critical medical anthropology that exemplify and extend its theoretical and empirical dimensions. Books in the series address topics across the broad range of subjects addressed by medical anthropologists and other scholars and practitioners working at the intersections of social science and medicine.

Volume 1
Global Warming and the Political Ecology of Health: Emerging Crises and Systemic Solutions, Hans Baer and Merrill Singer

Volume 2
The Healthy Ancestor: Embodied Inequality and the Revitalization of Native Hawaiian Health, Juliet McMullin

Volume 3
Drug Effects: Khat in Biocultural and Socioeconomic Perspective, Lisa L. Gezon

Volume 4
Syndemic Suffering: Social Distress, Depression, and Diabetes among Mexican Immigrant Women, Emily Mendenhall

SYNDEMIC SUFFERING

Social Distress, Depression, and Diabetes among
Mexican Immigrant Women

Emily Mendenhall

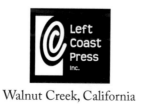

Walnut Creek, California

LEFT COAST PRESS, INC.
1630 North Main Street, #400
Walnut Creek, CA 94596
http://www.LCoastPress.com

ISBN 978-1-61132-141-8 hardcover
ISBN 978-1-61132-143-2 institutional electronic
ISBN 978-1-61132-683-3 consumer electronic

Library of Congress Cataloging-in-Publication Data:

Mendenhall, Emily, 1982–
   Syndemic suffering : social distress, depression, and diabetes among Mexican immigrant women / Emily Mendenhall.
      p. cm. — (Advances in critical medical anthropology ; v. 4)
   Includes bibliographical references.
ISBN 978-1-61132-141-8 (hardback : alk. paper) — ISBN 978-1-61132-143-2 (institutional ebook) — ISBN 978-1-61132-683-3 (consumer ebook)
   1. Diabetes in women. 2. Mexican American women—Health and hygiene.
   3. Mexican American women—Social conditions. I. Title.
      RA645.D5M46 2012
      362.1964'6200896872—dc23
                              2012020773

Printed in the United States of America

∞™ The paper used in this publication meets the minimum requirements of American National Standard for Information Sciences—Permanence of Paper for Printed Library Materials, ANSI/NISO Z39.48–1992.

Cover design by Piper Wallis
Cover photograph by Meredith Zielke. Mother + Child mural on Ashland Ave by Jeff Zimmerman (ca. 2001)

CONTENTS

Acknowledgments, 7

Introduction, 11

1

Synthesizing the Syndemic, 27

2

Synergies of the Self: The Endurance of Syndemic Suffering, 35

3

Unpacking VIDDA: An Analysis of Social Stress, 53

4

Borderlands: Immigration, Integration, and Isolation, 81

5

Narrative to Mechanism: Understanding Distress and Diabetes, 93

Conclusion, 107

Notes, 115

References, 121

Index, 139

About the Author, 145

ACKNOWLEDGMENTS

In dedication to María, and the rest of the women I met throughout the course of this project, and to Liz, and the rest of the staff committed to providing equitable health care in Cook County.

There is no way to sum up my gratitude for all those who have supported me throughout the years that culminated in this book.

The extraordinary openness of the women who shared their life stories with me inspired every page. I am forever humbled by their willingness to share such intimate and difficult aspects of their lives. I am motivated by their resilience to life's challenges. And I will forever be appreciative of their thoughtful (unsolicited) marriage advice.

This project would have been impossible without the unremitting support and guidance from Elizabeth Jacobs. Since I walked into her fourteenth-floor office in the fall of 2006 until I finished my last day of fieldwork, Liz has been the most incredible guide, teacher, and friend. Everyone deserves such a mentor.

This book would not have come to fruition without the support of Merrill Singer and Pamela Erickson. I am grateful for their confidence in my research, Merrill's critique of the manuscript, and more broadly for their contributions to the field of critical medical anthropology. I am equally indebted to senior editor Jennifer Collier who believed in this book from the beginning; few editors are as supportive, motivating, and knowledgeable about medical anthropology and global health as she.

Every book project benefits from many supportive people along the way. This research would not have been completed without the financial support from the National Science Foundation, Cells to Society at the Institute for Policy Research of Northwestern University, and The Graduate School at Northwestern University. Deborah Winslow, Eliza Earle, Katie Clarke-Myers, Tracy Tohtz,

Susan Higgins, and Dana Adam Fuller made grant application and management navigable. Elizabeth Jacobs provided me with an office and logistical support for this study. Veronica Hernandez Delgado patiently introduced me to the intricacies of conducting research at Cook County. Working in the General Medicine Clinic would have been difficult without the support of the nurses and clerks, and specifically of clinical administrator Eular Brown. There were many instances when my administrative friends came to the rescue, including Funeka, Audrean, Manju, Pawal, George, and Francisco, and I am thankful to Maria and Terry for their assistance with transcriptions. Finally, Sam del Pozo was an invaluable friend and resource when navigating the complexities of the Cook County system seemed impossible.

I am grateful for so many mentors and friends from my first intellectual home at the Rollins School of Public Health at Emory University. Forever, as I think critically about global health problems, the voice of Stan Foster will come to mind. I am a better medical anthropologist as a result of the endless encouragement from and intellectual exchange with my Emory community of friends, including Peter J. Brown, Sarah Willen, Erin Finley, Jennifer Kuzara, Kenneth Maes, Brandon Kohrt, Ryan Brown, Jed Stevenson, Svea Closser, Sarah Raskin, and Christine Murphy.

The Northwestern University Department of Anthropology provided me with deep intellectual roots. Rebecca Seligman read more drafts of my work in my first two years than is required of any advisor. Our dialogue shaped my understanding of the intersection of mind and body and provided many moments of clarity. Thomas McDade and Bill Leonard provided unfailing support and always encouraged me to wedge my work into the intersection of biological and cultural subfields. Jeff Huang tutored me in pipetting and guided me through the Human Biology Laboratory. Conversations with my cohort pushed me to think more broadly and deeply than I ever conceived. John Millhauser will forever be my teacher and good friend.

I will always have deep respect and gratitude for Jean O'Mahoney. Jean guided me through the waters of traumatic experience, distress, and chronic illness, and provided me not only with guidance as I wadded through women's stories but also with emotional clarity as I learned how to create space between the researcher and research. I have no idea how I could have done this project without her coaching around the delicate nature of working with people who have suffered so deeply.

My family and close friends are my rock, and I carry them with me always. Everyone should be so lucky to have as incredibly supportive, curious, and loving parents as I do. They read drafts, provided unfailing support and encouragement, and offered meals and a quiet haven for writing. My sister Kate lovingly bestowed sage advice and unending support. My brother-in-law Zach advised me on the experience of the family practitioner and provided important insight into the conclusion. My aunt Abby filled my belly and soul every Sunday. My husband supported me through every step of this project, be it via satellite phone from a rural village in South Sudan or Bihar, India. Adam, I am a happier, more balanced, and better person thanks to you.

Thank you.

INTRODUCTION

"The diabetes was probably [from] bad eating habits that I acquired from my whole family. But the heart disease I got, I always say people have broken my heart. So it broke." I met Marcía[1] as she sat in the waiting room of the primary care clinic at the old Cook County Hospital, reading a book and waiting to meet with her doctor. She wore a frayed white button-down blouse with baggy jeans and neon pink lipstick. Her graying dark hair was pulled back. Spun in an emotional three-hour narrative, Marcía revealed a life tapestry of poverty, childhood sexual abuse, severe depression, traumatic memories, suicide attempts, and the stress of managing multiple chronic illnesses, including type 2 diabetes, heart disease, and fibromyalgia.

Like many of the first- and second-generation Mexican immigrant women in my study, Marcía spoke intensely about struggles from her social and family life, focusing a great deal on her childhood. The transition from a childhood of work in the agricultural fields to full-time middle school in Chicago had been difficult. At the age of seventeen she married a man fourteen years her elder, her father's "drinking buddy," and had her first child at eighteen: "I wanted to get out of the house so I married him," she explained. After six years of marriage she left him because she believed that he was too controlling and "emotionally abusive"; she thought, "You're not treating me like that."

But leaving the marriage required incredible strength. As a child she had observed her father beating her mother, calling her names, and neglecting her needs. He had also sexually abused Marcía repeatedly between the ages of seven and seventeen, and these memories still haunted her. "I relive everything all the time. I think I'm seven years old 'cause I can remember like [it was] yesterday." During her adolescence she "was always trying to commit suicide" and had "two nervous breakdowns":

It wasn't until I got married when all those ideas stopped [. . .] After I had married and left, I said [to my sisters] don't—don't—don't put yourself in a position where you and Dad are alone. You know, we tried really hard, but he managed to get all of us and we had no control after we left. And you know, my mother would do nothing. She was as afraid of him as we were, so there was nothing that we could do about it. So we just waited until we could run. [Laughter] And we did.

When I asked Marcía if she was close with her nine siblings, she said, "It's hard because, you know, everybody's sick now. As we get older, everybody's sick." Most had diabetes and other physical health problems, and all of them struggled with depression and other manifestations of psychological distress. Two years before I met her, Marcía's youngest sister committed suicide. After that, Marcía and a sister organized a counseling session for all of the remaining siblings and they spoke openly of the abuse, most of them for the first time.

To readers unfamiliar with the field, Marcía's case may seem extreme. But her narrative is typical among the life stories collected for this book. Two out of every three of these first- and second-generation Mexican immigrant women with type 2 diabetes revealed that they had experienced some form of interpersonal abuse. More than half experienced physical abuse and almost one in four reported sexual abuse, often during childhood. Although gender-based violence is of growing concern in the United States, such high rates of abuse are uncommon in the general population (Briere and Elliot 2003). Recent scholarship indicates that Mexican immigrant populations report higher rates of abuse compared to populations in Mexico, and the incidence of abuse is higher still among those who are low-income second-, third-, and fourth-generation immigrant Mexican Americans (Holman, Silver, and Waitzkin 2000; Lown and Vega 2001; Heilemann, Kury, and Lee 2005; Baker et al. 2009). Scholars opine that the escalation of gender-based violence among the poor in the United States parallels increasing wealth disparities, festering in urban ghettos and correlating with the decline of social services and women's health (Harvey 2005; Bourgois 2009; Maskovsky and Susser 2009).

In the course of my research I realized that the social and psychological suffering women revealed through their life stories could provide insight into the clustering of depression and diabetes among poor Mexican immigrants and their families. Because the traditional biomedical approach that considers diabetes alone and detached from social contexts cannot encompass this reality (Singer and Clair 2003), I use a syndemic model to deconstruct such complex interactions. The term *syndemic* combines "synergy" and "epidemic" to conceptualize the intersection of multiple epidemics, including both diseases and epidemic social problems such as poverty. Merrill Singer first proposed the syndemics construct in the mid-1990s, and since then interest in syndemics has expanded greatly and across diverse disciplines, from anthropology to public health, nursing, psychology, dentistry, and biomedicine.

A syndemics framework describes situations in which adverse social conditions, such as poverty and oppressive social relationships, stress a population, weaken its natural defenses, and expose it to a cluster of interacting diseases (Singer 1996; Singer and Clair 2003; Singer et al. 2006; Singer 2009a, 2009b, 2011; Singer et al. 2011). The clustering and interaction of depression and diabetes is an exemplar case to study syndemic interactions, as these two diseases abide by three rules implicit in syndemic theory: the clustering of two diseases exists within a specific population; fundamental contextual and social factors are co-constructed with that cluster; and the disease cluster creates the potential for adverse disease interaction, increasing the burden of impacted populations. Thus, examining the syndemic interactions between diabetes and depression provides a model for the analysis of how disease clustering may be historically situated, socially driven, and co-constructed.

I have coined the term VIDDA Syndemic to illustrate the five core dimensions of health and social well-being among the immigrant women suffering from diabetes with whom I worked. *Violence* encompasses structural, symbolic, and everyday forms. *Immigration*-related stress results from the experience of migration, the fear of deportation once arrived in the U.S., and the feeling of social isolation that follows the loss of existing social networks. *Depression* is a chronic disorder for which very few poor women in the United States receive treatment, and in many cases described here it has been prolonged and internalized for decades. Type 2 *diabetes* is what unites the women in this study, although they may have myriad illnesses (indeed, insulin resistance both fuels and responds to the breakdown of the body). Finally, interpersonal *abuse* encompasses the salience of verbal, emotional, physical, and sexual abuse in women's life stories.

By evaluating these five key dimensions of VIDDA both as they are individually experienced and as they interact within VIDDA Syndemic theory, this book aims at demonstrating how increasing wealth disparity within our globalized, neoliberal[2] world contributes to the profoundly disparate distribution of burdensome chronic diseases among the poor. This chapter introduces some of the core concepts of this work: first, I discuss the inescapable influence of political economy on health and define three key forms of violence that play a central role in narratives like Marcía's: structural violence, symbolic violence, and everyday violence. Second, I describe the emergence of type 2 diabetes as a major health concern globally and within the United States specifically, in particular among ethnically and economically marginalized populations. Third, I introduce epidemiological and biological intersections between comorbid diabetes and depression that magnify the negative health impacts of these diseases. I then discuss why the syndemic approach is preferable to narrow, disease-focused approaches to epidemics and comorbidity, and elucidate the five key aspects of the VIDDA Syndemic.

Model of understanding health status- & include biological like syndemic social power, & #

The Political Economy of Health

For those who struggle each day to feed their families, maintain a safe and secure roof above their children's heads, and participate in the local and inevitably global economy, everyday life can be stressful. Understanding the complexities of the causes and consequences of such stress on the health and social well-being of marginalized and impoverished groups is a central goal of medical anthropology. Medical anthropology, and particularly biocultural and critical medical anthropology, insist that disease and suffering are as much social as they are biological. Biocultural anthropologists examine how political-economic and sociocultural changes impact human biology; critical medical anthropologists consider how macrosocial factors such as social inequality shape disease and suffering. Syndemics attend to both the "big picture" of health and to the synergistic interactions between social-psychological, social-biological, and psychological-biological domains (see Singer 2004a).

Medical anthropologists emphasize the role of violence, in its visible and less visible forms, as a key factor in health inequality (Kleinman, Das, and Lock 1996; Scheper-Hughes and Bourgois 2004; Rylko-Bauer, Whiteford, and Farmer 2009; Singer and Hodge 2010). While the consequences of visible violence on the health of those living through war and conflict are clear, the enduring legacies of invisible violence, such as Marcía's early experiences of extreme poverty and child abuse, are more difficult to measure, and can manifest themselves in the mind and body months, and often years, later. In other words, although less visible than acts of war, these "invisible" forms of violence also can have, as Carolyn Nordstrom noted, "a tomorrow" (2004, 224).

Three forms of violence discussed in the medical anthropology literature—structural, symbolic, and everyday violence—are important for understanding health disparities in high-income countries like the United States, and they frame my analysis of the social and political-economic inequities and individual traumas that contribute to the poor mental and physical health among socially disadvantaged women. I lay out these three modes separately to demonstrate how multiple layers of violence shape women's lives. However, the borders of structural, symbolic, and everyday violence are porous, and the interactions among them frequently compound the effects of any one of these forms of violence.

trying to alleviate suffering by distributing equal resources.

Sense of social justice

emphasis on valuing poor + middle class rather than wealthy power

Structural Violence

Stemming from the intellectual roots of Marxism and liberation theology, the concept of structural violence refers to the political-economic and social inequalities that can be both cause and consequence of poor mental and physical health (Galtung 1969; Farmer 1997; Bourgois 2001, 2009; Farmer 2004; Farmer et al. 2006). Structural violence becomes visible in the hegemony of institutions and ideologies and in the unequal trade between high- and low-income countries that sculpt the everyday experience of Mexican immigrants. Discrimination in the legal and social spheres, gender inequality, and racism also become visible forms of such violence (Bourgois 2009). In Marcía's case, the structural violence resides within a global economic structure that facilitated the devaluation of manual labor, fueling Marcía's family's need for increased income and thus Marcía's participation in migrant labor as a young girl. Working in the transient agricultural fields and living in barracks likely subjected Marcía to health risks that are widespread among migrant farmers, including exposures to pesticides, lack of hygienic facilities in the fields, and overcrowding in labor camps (Holmes 2006). Also, such a transient lifestyle is responsible for the lack of accountable social networks, which is likely to have exacerbated her exposure to the oppressive relationship with her father (and his abuse). I will explore this problem in depth, because the breakdown of social networks and social protection is at the center of many women's stories of interpersonal abuse. Hence, I examine the violence that produces violence, emphasizing the relationship of structural violence to women's experiences of domestic abuse. As such, structural violence may be understood as a form of subjugation that is institutionalized and associated with health and social problems.

anthrop. movement to deliver ppl from communism

Scholars from biocultural anthropology and social epidemiology have documented how political-economic inequalities and increasing wealth disparity contribute to negative health outcomes among the socially disadvantaged (Singer et al. 1992; Dressler 1993; Singer 1994; Wilkinson 1996; Goodman and Leatherman 1998; Marmot and Wilkinson 2001; McDade 2002; Rock 2003; Wilkinson and Marmot 2003; Gravlee, Dressler, and Bernard 2005). Much of this scholarship focuses on how the stress that derives from structural inequalities functions as a major contributor to poor health. While these studies document how such inequality might "get under the skin," more research is needed that illuminates how larger structural factors figure into both microlevel social processes and the individual's emotional and physical health. I take this approach to reveal the vicious cycle by which the structural violence fundamental to our current political and economic system exacerbates distress and disease among socially disadvantaged populations.

income gap associated w/ health behavior

poorest ppl are most vulnerable, also includes shrinking middle class.

Symbolic Violence

The concept of symbolic violence was first introduced by Pierre Bourdieu (1989, 2001) and refers to the implicit inequities—such as sexism, racism, and classism—that exist in daily life and contribute significantly to poor health (Bourdieu 1989, 2001; Bourdieu and Wacquant 2004). Symbolic violence manifests itself in the ways individuals internalize the social domination to which they are subjected due to the gender, race, and class structures of their political-economic and social environments. Bourdieu and Wacquant argue that gender domination more than any other form shows that "symbolic violence accomplishes itself through an act of cognition and of misrecognition that lies beyond—or beneath—the controls of consciousness and will" (2004, 273). Marcía's perception as a teen that getting married and starting her own family were the only ways she could escape her abusive family situation is one example of how social constructions of gender can shape a woman's agency in making decisions (from a limited pool of bad options). However, this does not mean that symbolic violence prohibits or limits the agency of the individual to change her or his situation, as Marcía's case demonstrates: Marcía was determined not to reproduce the family life of her childhood and, unlike her mother, Marcía terminated her marriage when she saw signs of potential abuse. Marcía seemingly felt she had limited power over her personal situation, yet she was not without agency to address and transform negative circumstances.

The notion of symbolic violence also encompasses the "domination of the dominant by his domination" (Bourdieu and Wacquant 2004, 273). In the case of the patriarchal advantage of men, this means that men are dominated by cultural and social expectations of masculinity and subconsciously try to live up to the ideals of what it means to be a man. For example, the failure to uphold cultural ideals about masculinity publicly (as a wage earner) has been associated with the increase in male aggression in the private sphere (Singer et al. 1992; Singer 1997; Bourgois 2009). In this sense, the social construction of what it means to be a man (and, specifically, a Mexican man in Chicago) may contribute to coping mechanisms and compensating behaviors like alcoholism, drug abuse, or domestic abuse, as men struggle to fit into an expected familial role as Mexican patriarchs that is unrealistic in contemporary political-economic contexts (Gutmann 1999; Hirsch 2003a). Indeed, such unbalanced structures force us to move beyond feminist notions of men as independent perpetrators of violence against women and instead examine how individuals negotiate their own roles of dominator and dominated within a larger political-economic and social system. *gender role of men that dominate women, both have negative roles in their society.*

bi-directional effect

Everyday Violence

Although intimately tied to structural violence and symbolic violence, gender-based violence captures a particular kind of "everyday" or "normalized" violence against women. While structural violence deals with political-economic inequality and symbolic violence deals with internalized sociocultural expectations, everyday violence refers to those acts of violence against women and children that are repeated so often in everyday life that, over time, they become routine (Scheper-Hughes 1992; Bourgois 1998; Bourgois, Prince, and Moss 2004; Bourgois 2009). In other words, socially unacceptable acts, such as wife battering or child mistreatment, when kept hidden and unaddressed over the long term, may become part of an individual's everyday experience, and in this sense, become almost normalized. Indeed, the routine nature of Marcía's father's sexual abuse exemplifies this form of normalized violence: a systematic pattern of abuse to which many turned a blind eye.

Epidemiological studies reveal that women more commonly report having experienced child sexual abuse than men, and children of immigrants report higher rates of childhood sexual abuse compared to immigrants themselves (Baker et al. 2005; Heilemann, Kury, and Lee 2005; Baker et al. 2009). These acts of violence are particularly insidious because the mistreatment takes place in the home, away from the public, and often is kept between the perpetrator and these most vulnerable victims. As a result such violence remains invisible—the victim has no voice, no advocate, and limited means to escape, and is thus forced to function within the context of such everyday violence.

The Emergence of Diabetes

As Melanie Rock argues, "it is worthwhile to consider how epidemics achieve social significance, both through their material presence and through the symbolic representation of their causes and effects" (2003, 155). Type 2 diabetes mellitus (also referred to as adult-onset and non-insulin-dependent diabetes mellitus; hereafter, "diabetes") is a good example of a disease that has achieved social significance and is clearly linked to increasingly urban lifestyles and social inequalities. Clinically diabetes, measured by insulin resistance, is known to result from obesity and a sedentary lifestyle and has been associated even with various factors such as viral infection and food-borne toxins. Scholars describe diabetes as the disease of "modernization" because of the strong relationships between economic development and urbanization, particular lifestyles (diet and activity patterns), stress, psychological distress, and dissolution of social networks, all of which function as major contributors to obesity, diabetes's greatest risk factor (McGarvey et al. 1989; Stunkard and Sorensen 1993; Zimmet, Alberti, and Shaw 2001; Lieberman 2003). However, the intersections of these factors with political-economic *inequalities* are not always recognized.

On a global scale, obesity and diabetes have risen exponentially over the past thirty years. In 1985, diabetes affected around 30 million adults, increasing five-fold to approximately 151 million adults (4.6 percent of the 20–79 age group) by 2000. In 2010, the adults suffering from diabetes were around 285 million, or approximately 6.6 percent of the adult population. Estimates for 2030 show the number ballooning to 438 million adults (7.8 percent) worldwide (International Diabetes Federation 2009). The largest percentage of the global population with diabetes resides in China, India, and the United States. The International Diabetes Federation projects that the number of people living with diabetes will escalate in these countries, as well as in other emerging economies that resemble the fast-paced modernization observed in China and India. Particularly at risk are women and people between the ages of forty and fifty-nine.

Curious global patterns of diabetes distribution provide some insight into the role played by political-economic and social processes in the diabetes problem. For example, low-income countries, such as much of sub-Saharan Africa, show the lowest incidence of diabetes among the global population. In these economies, diabetes afflicts primarily women and individuals living in urban centers with the financial security to lead more Western-oriented lifestyles, characterized by higher caloric diets and reduced physical activity (BeLue et al. 2009; Dalal et al. 2011). Diabetes is expected to spread in low-income countries in tandem with economic development, as it has already in middle-income countries such as Brazil, Mexico, and India (Popkin et al. 2009). Within these countries, wealth inequalities play an important role in the distribution of non-communicable diseases, such as diabetes, and communicable diseases, such as tuberculosis—a phenomenon described as the double burden of disease (Subramanian, Kawachi, and Davey Smith 2007). In the past, diabetes clustered primarily among affluent groups. However, recent epidemiological studies reveal a socioeconomic reversal of diabetes, as lower-income groups are showing higher incidence of insulin resistance (Monteiro et al. 2004). Examination of the diabetes prevalence within high-income countries like the United States, therefore, provides insight into what might happen within these emerging economies. In particular, studies on the emergence of diabetes in North America indicate that diabetes is one of the ways in which social suffering becomes embodied in the experience of socially disadvantaged groups (Rock 2003; Mendenhall et al. 2010).

As the seventh leading cause of death in the United States, diabetes is an established public health threat and medical problem. National surveillance of diabetes indicates that the disease has been escalating steadily in the United States since the late 1950s. In 1958 the percentage of people with diabetes in the United States was 0.93 percent, compared to 1.62 percent in 1968, 2.37 percent in 1978, 2.56 percent in 1988, 3.90 percent in 1998, and 6.29 percent in 2008 (International Diabetes Federation 2009). The most rapid increases in diabetes prevalence are found in tandem with the most rapid expansions of wealth inequality. In the twenty-year period between 1981 and 2001, when wealth inequality in the United States increased dramatically (Keister and Moller 2000), there were significantly correlated ($ß = 0.81$; $p < 0.05$)[3] increases in family income inequality (measured by the Gini coefficient, which marks the difference between the highest and lowest wage earners) and diabetes prevalence (Johnson, Smeeding, and Boyle Torrey 2005; Centers for Disease Control and Prevention 2010). Figure 1 illustrates these parallel trends between escalating wealth inequality and diabetes prevalence.

Complicating this trend line is the fact that escalating rates of diabetes in the United States were not distributed equally among the population, and today wide variations in diabetes prevalence persist among ethnic groups. For example, lifetime risk for diabetes among Hispanic women is estimated to be as high as 52.5 percent, compared to 31.2 percent lifetime risk among white women.

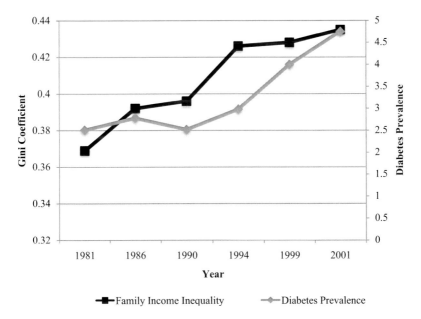

Figure 1 Twenty-year trends of increasing income inequality and diabetes prevalence in the United States

Hispanic men's lifetime risk for diabetes, however, is lower than the risk for women, at 45.6 percent, but similarly higher than the risk of white male counterparts, at 26.7 percent (Narayan et al. 2003). Such high rates of diabetes are unsurprising given that one in three adults in the United States are obese regardless of age or ethnicity, and that women and Mexican Americans are significantly more likely to be obese when compared to the general population (Ogden et al. 2006).

Perhaps of greatest concern is the national surveillance data that reveal diabetes incidence is increasing among Mexican Americans, surpassing groups with the highest prevalence, such as African Americans and Puerto Ricans (Centers for Disease Control and Prevention 2010).[4] A recent analysis of the 1999–2002 NHANES data reveals diabetes prevalence to be much higher among Mexican Americans compared to the general population in all age categories (Cowie et al. 2010). For example, among individuals between the ages of forty and fifty-nine, Mexican American diabetes prevalence was 11.5 percent compared to 6.6 percent in the general population. This disparity is maintained with age: 25 percent of Mexican Americans over the age of sixty-five were diagnosed with diabetes compared to 15.1 percent of the general population (ibid). While Mexican American women were slightly more likely to develop diabetes at a younger age than men, diabetes prevalence among older Mexican Americans did not vary by gender (ibid). These data bring forth questions about the ways in which macrosocial forces frame social contexts that contribute to such disease burden.

Diabetes and Depression Comorbidity

Concurrent or comorbid depression among Mexican Americans is increasing along with the rise in diabetes prevalence and is extremely high: around one quarter of individuals within this population who have diabetes also report symptoms of depression (de Groot et al. 2006; Li et al. 2008). This estimation is almost double for Mexican Americans with diabetes over the age of sixty-five, and more women with diabetes (58 percent) are affected than are men with diabetes (40 percent) (Black, Markides, and Ray 2003). Depression among people with diabetes is particularly troubling because depression is associated with hyperglycemia, which in turn increases the likelihood of macrovascular complications, such as cardiovascular disease and high blood pressure, and microvascular complications, such as retinopathy, neuropathy, and nephropathy (de Groot et al. 2001). While the rates of acute depression are similar across ethnic groups in the United States, disability and death related to chronic depression, limited access to mental health care, and diabetes complications more often affect Mexican Americans and women compared to whites and men, respectively (Anderson et al. 2001; Black, Markides, and Ray 2003; de Groot et al. 2006; Gonzalez et al. 2010).

Epidemiologists and clinical investigators have largely focused on how the debilitating and distressing aspects of diabetes contribute to depression. However, in the past decade a growing body of research has documented a bidirectional relationship between diabetes and depression, suggesting that depression is both a consequence of and a contributor to diabetes (Talbot and Nouwen 2000; Musselman et al. 2003; Knol et al. 2006; Golden et al. 2007; Golden et al. 2008; Mezuk et al. 2008; Egede and Ellis 2010). As a result, there have been recent calls for more studies that examine how social distress may contribute to depression among people with diabetes and, in turn, how this might contribute to diabetes onset, morbidity, and mortality (Fisher et al. 2001; Rock 2003; Fisher et al. 2008; Pouwer, Kupper, and Adriaanse 2010).

Clinical and epidemiological studies have mostly maintained a biomedical focus on investigations of "causality" and "comorbidity" between these diseases, with little attention to the structural, social, and emotional forces that may interact synergistically with diabetes and depression and contribute to their co-occurrence. As such, a great deal of research has been invested into studies of why people with diabetes are two times more likely to be depressed than the general population, emphasizing the role of diabetes as the *cause* of depression in this population (Anderson et al. 2001; Li et al. 2009). There is also increasing interest in the role of depression and, even more broadly, psychosocial stress as cause of or risk factor for diabetes (Fisher et al. 2001; Fisher et al. 2008; Golden et al. 2008; Pan et al. 2010; Pouwer, Kupper, and Adriaanse 2010). However, few studies have adequately represented the complexity of such distress. For instance, none of these studies considers how historical, social, emotional, and biological factors may synergistically interact to perpetuate these parallel and interactive epidemics.

Syndemics Theory

The syndemics orientation departs from traditional biomedical approaches that treat diseases as distinct entities, detached from the social contexts of their carriers (Singer and Clair 2003). Historically, disease-focused approaches proved useful in focusing medical attention on the immediate causes and biological expressions of disease. This orientation has largely shaped the course of biomedicine, as clinicians often focus on the physical aspects of disease without exploring social and emotional factors. Yet, just as culturally defined syndromes are situated within cultural and historical contexts, so too biomedical constructions of disease are culturally and historically contingent (Good 1994). The syndemics framework requires the medical community to take a step back from its focus on disease as a singular, self-contained entity and requires investigators and clinicians to consider how social and psychological factors synergistically interact with physical health.

Syndemics theory has been used to address a wide range of synergistic interactions, from historical interpretations of the global influenza pandemic of 1918 to present-day interactions between HIV/AIDS and malnutrition in sub-Saharan Africa (Singer 2009a).[5] The first syndemic proposed by Singer (1996) was called the SAVA Syndemic and modeled a critical triangulation of substance abuse, violence, and AIDS among low-income Puerto Ricans in the United States. His argument was founded on the notion that the AIDS epidemic was inextricably linked with a social context characterized by poverty, low rates of education and employment, and concurrent alcoholism, which together fueled youth participation in gang activity, drug trade, and violence. Through the triangulation of these three dynamic problems, Singer's syndemic theory emphasized how the clustering of substance abuse and AIDS was the corollary of social context.

Understanding the role of social problems in disease clustering requires distinguishing between the syndemic interactions of two diseases and the notion of comorbidity. As Mustanski and colleagues explain, "comorbidity research tends to focus on the nosological issues of boundaries and overlap of diagnoses, while syndemic research focuses on communities experiencing co-occurring epidemics that additively increase negative health consequences" (2007, 39). For example, Rosa González-Guarda and colleagues (2011) contend that mental health problems are intrinsic to the spread of HIV and AIDS among Hispanics in the United States and therefore must be incorporated into interpretations of the SAVA Syndemic for this group. They argue that mental distress seems to stem from social factors associated with immigration to the United States, including separation from family and social networks, labor demands, and shifting gender roles, all of which are critical conduits of HIV risk (Gonzalez-Guarda, Florom-Smith, and Thomas 2011). If we overlook the role of mental distress within the triangulation of SAVA within this group, we may overlook important individual-level factors that facilitate behaviors that increase the risk to develop AIDS. Furthermore, by interconnecting depression and HIV through social and behavioral pathways, this syndemic framework provides a more holistic interpretation for clinicians and social workers working with immigrant Latinos in the U.S., as opposed to comorbidity.

The syndemics approach provides a much needed intellectual and political shift that has the potential to influence the ways in which Americans conceive of and treat health problems. The National Institutes of Health and the

Centers for Disease Control and Prevention have already shown interest in the syndemics approach, calling for studies rooted in this integrated, multifaceted perspective (Singer 2009a). Yet, to date, few scholars have focused on syndemics among women, and the research presented here is the second extensive study of syndemics thus far.

The VIDDA Syndemic

The acronym *VIDDA* (in Spanish, *vida* is "life") communicates an interactive framework that analyzes social contexts as intrinsic to the clustering of depression and diabetes among Mexican immigrant women in Chicago. As I noted earlier in this introduction, VIDDA incorporates the syndemic interactions of *V*iolence (structural, symbolic, and everyday), *I*mmigration (stress and social isolation), *D*epression, *D*iabetes, and *A*buse (verbal, emotional, physical, and sexual). The acronym "VIDDA" echoes a familiar dictum repeated by many of the women interviewed for this study: *la vida es dura* (life is hard). Cultural anthropologist Roger Lancaster similarly employed this maxim to capture the intense suffering and resilience of his interlocutors in his book *Life is Hard: Machismo, Danger, and the Intimacy of Power in Nicaragua* (1994). His interpretation of the dictum describes the depth of struggle encompassed in the VIDDA Syndemic:

> A coda set to the rhythm of life's frustrations, this maxim can relate the *duress* of social and economic crisis experienced as personal conditions. It marks, too, the *duration* of the crisis that renders life so very hard. Its pessimism, its fatalism, can plainly serve as a sort of alibi, an excuse, that relieves the individual speaker of the consequences of his own actions . . . This proverb can bring to light the strength and *endurance* of the people who survive life's hardships. It marks, by turn, the banality of suffering, the intimacy of power, the comfort of resignation, and the resilience of the oppressed. (Lancaster 1994, xvi)

Lancaster suggests that the capillaries of power that permeate individualized suffering also shape people's responses to the duress of their distress. In the midst of such suffering, then, the maxim "life is hard" reveals people's resilience to such hardship. Indeed, Marcía's case exemplifies the possibility of maintaining resilience amidst repeated challenges. In this sense, her life story cannot be interpreted apart from her early childhood abuse anymore than from her struggles with chronic depression and diabetes. Nor can Marcía's ability to overcome such adversities and persevere to protect her daughter and her family from the aftermath of violence be detached from her life story. Yet, despite her resilience and perseverance in the face of a hard life, the duress and duration of life's stresses are inscribed in her depression and diabetes. Thus, the VIDDA Syndemic shows how various dimensions of social, emotional, and biological stresses, which are experienced often as a single multifaceted force, make life so very hard.

In many ways, VIDDA Syndemic theory parallels the embodiment construct proposed by social epidemiologist Nancy Krieger. Krieger argues, "We literally incorporate, biologically, the material and social world in which we live" (2005, 352). Embodiment is a process and construct that integrates soma, psyche, and society. Krieger contends that disease can be understood to be a clue to life histories, hidden and revealed, and a reminder of the consequences of diverse forms of inequality (Krieger 1999, 2005). Like syndemics theory, the embodiment construct values social, psychological, and biological aspects of disease—an approach that is too often absent from biomedicine—and describes how deleterious environments, social inequalities, and emotional distresses manifest themselves, and can be measured, in the body.

Such notions of embodiment are central to the VIDDA Syndemic. In Marcía's case, her depression and diabetes are not only the consequence of a hard life, but they are also consequences of one another, and causes of ongoing emotional and social suffering. The actual biological interactions between depression and diabetes will be explored in depth in chapter 5, but here it is important to state that the biological interaction between the two diseases also contributes to syndemic clustering within this population. As such, this study of diabetes does not consider the disease to be an endpoint, or "outcome," as it is in biomedicine, but rather considers the significance of glycemic control to be one measure of a stressful life. Treating diabetes as the "outcome" leads clinicians, social workers, and investigators to focus on the physical aspects of individual diseases rather than on the social and emotional causes or consequences of suffering.

Thus, the VIDDA Syndemic emphasizes the role of social forces, such as feelings of social detachment and interpersonal abuse, and structural and symbolic forces, such as violence and subjugation, in promoting the clustering and interaction of diabetes and depression. For instance, Marcía's narrative ties her suffering to chronic adversities of poverty, sexual abuse, emotional mistreatment, and lack of social and institutional support that shaped her personal experience and continue to interact with her chronic diseases. The VIDDA Syndemic models these multiple levels of suffering as an interactive system through which individualized narratives of social, psychological, and physical distress can be understood. While based on the lived experiences of first- and second-generation Mexican immigrant women with diabetes in Chicago, the interactions found in the VIDDA Syndemic will likely provide insight into the burden of depression and diabetes afflicting women living in other contexts of heightened psychological and social suffering throughout the Americas.

Chapter Overview

Chapter 1 begins with a brief discussion of the complexities of conducting research with women who have suffered from a history of interpersonal abuse and confront chronic mental and physical health problems. I then introduce the women of "Mexican Chicago" who are the focus of this book. These women are among the poorest residents of Chicago and seek diabetes care at the city's largest public hospital clinic. Finally, I describe how I triangulated life history narrative and social, psychiatric, and biological data in order to generate VIDDA Syndemic theory.

In chapter 2 I investigate how individuals use narratives to make sense of the connections between personal suffering and diabetes, and why narratives are useful tools for developing syndemics theory. I illustrate the syndemic interactions fundamental to VIDDA Syndemic theory through two women's life stories, which present some of the most extreme forms of social distress I encountered in my research. The first is the story of Domenga, a Mexican immigrant who has endured a great deal of psychological and social suffering, such as poverty, undocumented migration to Chicago, rape in early adulthood, the loss of her husband to a work accident, chronic and untreated depression, and diabetes. Second is the story of Rosie, a second-generation Mexican American who was raped and kidnapped during childhood and largely internalized this experience until her late-adult diabetes diagnosis. Through her diagnosis and access to the safety-net health system, Rosie opened up about the childhood abuse for the first time. I analyze these life stories to demonstrate the five key dimensions of VIDDA Syndemic theory and to introduce the reader to the lived lives of the women in this study.

Chapter 3 presents the major forms of social stresses that are at the heart of the VIDDA Syndemic. I situate this chapter within critical medical anthropology's long-standing critique of biomedicine and of what Paul Farmer has called "immodest claims of causality" (1999, 4). I do so to underscore the problem of overemphasizing cultural and psychological explanations of disease, which can result in an oversight of the deeply troubling contextual and structural problems that are fundamental to the stress-diabetes interface. Then, I systematically unpack nine common stressful experiences that women described in their life history narratives, including: interpersonal abuse, health problems, family issues, loss of a family member, immigration, work stress, financial troubles, neighborhood violence, and feelings of social isolation. Based on my analysis of women's life stories, I determine these stresses to be core mediators of the stress-diabetes interface for Mexican immigrant women in Chicago.

In chapter 4 I focus in particular on immigration stress and the role of social integration in the VIDDA Syndemic. In the past twenty years, anthropologists and health scientists have become concerned with the deterioration of immigrants' health after their arrival in the United States. This chapter introduces both the scholarly dialogue surrounding this phenomenon and the established anthropological critique of focusing on "culture" as the primary vehicle for transforming health behaviors and associated disease trends. I scrutinize the life history narratives to illustrate how immigration experiences figure into women's life stories and to understand the role of immigration in the reporting of the nine narrative themes presented in chapter 3. After introducing the tragic circumstances of Mari's immigration story, I contend that the breakdown of social networks and resultant feelings of marginalization, which cannot be dissociated from the transformations of the global economic structure, are at the root of poor health within this population.

Chapter 5 turns to the numerous psychological, behavioral, and biological pathways that are central to the VIDDA Syndemic. Understanding the roles of these various pathways is essential to syndemic theory, as the relationship between depression and diabetes has biological underpinnings that go beyond the social or behavioral domains. I first describe the emergence of diabetes and discuss the factors that facilitate its onset. Then, I discuss how the cumulative effects of social stress throughout the life course can impact individuals and populations substantially and analyze six pathways through which depression and diabetes interact bidirectionally.

The conclusion returns to the synergistic interactions among distress, depression, and diabetes, and their impact on the lives of Mexican women in Chicago. I review how the syndemic framework provides a superior understanding of health, as opposed to a narrower focus on epidemics and comorbidities, because it incorporates mediating factors that singular or disease-oriented frameworks overlook. I further demonstrate how the narrative approach provides a unique window into the synergies of suffering faced by women in this study through Teresa's story. Teresa describes how a Spanish-speaking psychiatrist at the public hospital largely dismissed her social and emotional problems. In doing so, the doctor not only communicated that her problems were not stressful enough to receive psychological support, but he also failed to recognize how such stress might figure into her diabetes care. As long as the social and psychological aspects of people's suffering are overlooked, their synergies with chronic diseases like diabetes will continue. By recognizing synergies among these realms and providing integrated treatment that attends to these various facets of suffering, I believe there is possibility to curb syndemics among the poor.

1

SYNTHESIZING THE SYNDEMIC

Research on personal stress and traumatic experience can be tricky, particularly for a medical anthropologist untrained in clinical psychology and ill-equipped to provide psychological counseling. Marcía's opening vignette illustrates how attending to the stress-diabetes interface among Mexican immigrant women in Chicago often presented immense challenges associated with bearing witness to social and psychological suffering, from sexual violence to unremitting feelings of loneliness and fear of future chronic disease outcomes. Therefore, I devote this chapter to discussing the unique circumstances of the women I met throughout the course of this research and the challenges associated with interviewing them about the severe stress from their life histories. This chapter also describes how I came to recognize the complexities of the VIDDA Syndemic through a multilayered, mixed methodology.

María's story is typical. She immigrated to the United States as a young adult, created a new life for herself with her husband, started a family, and lived many years apart from her social network in Mexico. I first met María in 2007 when I was conducting exploratory ethnographic research, and at that time she revealed a complicated life history that intertwined difficult aspects from her past with ongoing stresses from her diabetes and family life. She disclosed a history of child sexual abuse, and like many other women expressed her struggles with the emotional and physical abuse associated with her husband's alcoholism. In her late fifties, this was the first time she had shared her childhood experience with anyone.

We met again three years later at the General Medicine Clinic (GMC) at the old Cook County Hospital where she was seeking care for her diabetes and depression. This was at the beginning of my research and I was happy to see her; we met with a warm embrace. At first I was surprised that she remembered me and seemed genuinely happy to see me. Although hugging my respondents after an intense interview had already become somewhat of a norm, such a reception after a number of years was obviously touching. I remembered vividly the exchange with María because it had been an incredibly powerful experience, and I assumed this was the reason she recognized me, as well. In fact, many of the narratives I collected in 2007 were ironed into my memory. I spent many months synthesizing that exploratory data and making sense of their experiences.

What was interesting about María's second interview was its inconsistency with the first. She had lost some weight and her depressive symptoms had diminished. After our first meeting, María had sought support from a counselor associated with the GMC and had worked through some of her emotional struggles. She also reported that her husband had passed away and she had moved into a garden apartment to live on her own for the first time. During that second exchange I was surprised that she did not bring up her experiences with childhood sexual abuse; in fact, when I asked if she had any stressful experiences from her past, she said there were memories that she wouldn't discuss and changed the subject. What was most interesting about this interview was that María indicated that she had no reason to share such struggles with me. This was the only exchange in which I faced such dismissal of some of the most difficult questions in my interview guide. I will never know if it was because she had worked through her emotional problems or felt as though she had shared too much with me already. However, the difference between the two interviews brought to light an important question. Were the high rates of interpersonal abuse reported in my study due to the fact that women rarely had an outlet to share their narratives of social and psychological suffering? Was our dialogue that outlet? In many cases, indeed, women stated that the interview was the first or second time they had ever fully disclosed their history of abuse.

Attending to the mental health of my interlocutors was a challenge because all but three women's life history narratives revealed one of the nine major stressors that are highlighted in chapter 3. I personally connected women who revealed a history of sexual abuse and severe symptoms of depression or post-traumatic stress disorder (PTSD) with the psychiatry department that was adjoined to the GMC. I was particularly determined to do so with the eight women who reported suicidal ideation, and followed up with the social worker at the GMC as well. In some cases, I called my interlocutor the following week to check in and make sure that she had followed up with a counselor. For personal care, an issue that is rarely addressed in anthropological scholarship (see Simmons and Koester 2003),

I found my own therapist to talk through women's narratives of suffering so that I would not internalize their stories and take them with me into my personal life. This is common in the field of clinical psychology and I believe that this type of self-care is critical for anthropologists working with populations who have suffered so deeply.

I worked onsite in this clinic for almost two years and was involved with a larger multiphase study on culture, diabetes, immigration, and health care for five years. I recruited women for this study from the GMC while they waited for their routine diabetes care appointments with their general internist. Like most public clinics, patients at the GMC wait for hours in a crowded room populated with people from all walks of life, often waiting at least two and sometimes up to six hours to see their physicians.

A wide variety of languages can be overheard in the GMC, from Spanish to Hindi and even some African dialects. Official interpreters for twelve languages are spread thin across the hospital, and the GMC alone serves more than 40,000 primary-care visits per year.[1] This is one of one hundred outpatient clinics associated with the 450-bed hospital. Serving the social and psychological needs of all of these patients at the time of this study were eight psychiatrists, two nurse practitioners, four nurses, and three psychologists.[2] The GMC and community-based clinics also often have a social worker on staff to meet the needs of their patients, and some employ an additional nurse counselor or psychologist. When this study was carried out, one bilingual Spanish-speaking social worker worked within the GMC itself and there were two physicians, one nurse, and three psychologists who were Spanish-speaking in the adjacent Psychiatry Department. Some clinicians and clerks at the GMC also spoke Spanish, but Spanish-speaking patients were not always paired with them. The unmet needs for Spanish-speaking diabetes care is evident in the fact that 25–30 percent of the patients at the GMC are Latino and 30–40 percent are diabetic.[3] Data on the nationalities of all Latino patients at the GMC are not available, but based on my experience recruiting for various research projects, I estimate that the percentage of people of Mexican descent among all Latinos seeking care at the GMC resemble those of the city at large (75 percent).

Many of these patients sincerely appreciate the care provided for them at the GMC and realize that they would be much worse off without it. Despite the many hours spent waiting for clinical care and then again in the pharmacy for medications, many of my interlocutors stated that they could not find a better doctor. My mentor, who worked at this clinic for twelve years, exemplifies the sort of physicians who dedicate their career to this population. She spent hours of valuable time on the phone with her patients, social services, and other hospital departments to ensure that her patients' needs were met. This is obviously not a lucrative profession in the medical world and presents unique challenges, but the senior attending physicians and long-standing nurses who devote their careers to this clinic are certainly dedicated to their patients. Nevertheless, many of my interlocutors expressed concern about the care they received as a result of the overburdened system and described the many challenges faced while seeking care in the public clinic, which I will discuss in depth in the conclusion.

Very few eligible women I approached declined to participate, most likely because they knew they had an extended wait to see their doctor and could spend that time speaking with me in a private room adjacent to the waiting room. The nurses were extremely accommodating and would notify the woman I was interviewing if it was time for her appointment, and oftentimes they would simply wedge them into the schedule after we had completed our interview. I think that some of the women participated in the interview because they were compensated for their time, which is customary for research at the GMC.[4] However, many of my interlocutors thanked me for listening to their stories after we completed the interview and I believe the majority truly enjoyed conversing for a couple hours about issues of keen personal interest to them. Indeed, many women stated that they found it cathartic, or in one woman's words: "I feel like I just had a therapy session!" In addition to the life history narratives, I collected information about diabetes duration,[5] diabetes severity[6] and distress,[7] diabetes management,[8] depression[9] and PTSD,[10] anthropometrics,[11] and finger-stick blood samples, which were used to evaluate diabetes control.[12]

The Women of Mexican Chicago

The term "Mexican Chicago" reflects the long-standing demographic, economic, and political presence of Mexicans in the city. In *Rancheros in* Chicagoacán (2006) Marcia Farr argues that the cultural and linguistic ties between Mexican communities in Chicago and Michoacán[13] are so interconnected that they can be understood to be one community named Chicagoacán. In *Working the Boundaries*, Nicholas De Genova deems "the production of Mexican Chicago a conjunctural space with transformative repercussions in all directions" (2005, 99). In this sense, De Genova understands Mexican Chicago to be inherently transnational and to provide a fluid exchange of goods, ideas, language, and people, influencing the social contexts in both Mexico and the United States. Indeed, it is impossible to discuss Mexicans in Chicago without recognizing the deep, multithreaded, and everyday bidirectional ties with various sending communities in Mexico.

The majority of Mexican immigration to Chicago involves "chain migration" in which people from one place in Mexico migrate to Chicago and petition for family and social networks to join them, resulting in localized movements (such as "Chicagoacán"). Although Mexican immigrants are known to immigrate in groups and move within their social networks, Mexican presence in Chicago defies the traditional image of Mexicans as a regional minority group (Farr 2006). The distinctness of Chicago as a city and Mexican immigrant Mecca lies in the "city's ethnic and industrial diversity, its Roman Catholicism, its neighborhood-oriented political and social life, and [since the 1950s] its unique combination of Latino populations" (Kerr 1976, 11). The historical legacy of Mexican Chicago has been described in depth elsewhere as a rich intercultural space with intimate, transgenerational ties with Mexico and concurrent struggles against discrimination and marginalization in Chicago (see Kerr 1976, 1977; Weber 1982; Portes and Bach 1985; Chock 1996; Valdes 2000; De Genova and Ramos-Zayas 2003; Arredondo and Vaillant 2004; De Genova 2005; Farr 2006; Arredondo 2008; De Genova and Peutz 2010; Montoya 2011).

Second in size only to Los Angeles in the United States, the greater Chicago area counts one million people of Mexican descent, with more than half a million living in Chicago itself (584,100 people) and making up 21.4 percent of the urban population (U.S. Census Bureau 2010). This population is not static but rather is a mixture of recent immigrants, children of immigrants, descendants of immigrants' children, and people with mixed parenthood. They come from a broad spectrum of Mexican states, different ethnicities, and varied educational backgrounds. Approximately one-quarter of this population lives below the poverty line (Bishaw and Iceland 2003). This book depicts women's experiences within that one-quarter of the Chicago Mexican population that struggles at or below the poverty line.

All of the 121 women interviewed for this book were between the ages of forty and sixty-five, self-identified as Mexican or Mexican American, and sought diabetes care at the GMC. Two-thirds of the women I interviewed were born in Mexico. Many of these first-generation Mexican immigrants had lived in Chicago for more than twenty-five years and had settled in one of the Mexican enclave neighborhoods, such as Pilsen or La Villita (Little Village). Very few of the first-generation immigrant women had ever been employed, and many lived with their children or in an apartment adjacent to one or more family members. Caregiving for grandchildren or other family members was commonly their full-time or part-time job. Most of these women spoke Spanish only (n = 63) and half were undocumented (n = 33). I categorized women born in the United States to Mexican immigrant parents and Mexican-born individuals who immigrated to the U.S. before the ages of seven or eight as second-generation Mexican immigrants. The majority of the second-generation Mexican American women I interviewed were bilingual,[14] had completed high school, technical training, or college, and had maintained jobs throughout their adult lives, although many were retired or on disability due to poor health. Most of these women lived with their partners or on their own in apartments in more ethnically diverse neighborhoods, such as South Chicago and Logan Square.

Nevertheless, these categories seemed somewhat arbitrary because there was a great deal of diversity in women's upbringings. Some women had spent much of their childhood living between border towns, such as Laredo, Texas, and Nuevo Laredo, Mexico. They crossed family and national borders with ease and led largely transnational, bicultural lives. Other women had spent much of their lives in Mexico, immigrating to Chicago only five to ten years before I met them to work as caregivers for their grandchildren or to seek comfort upon the death of a husband. Others had never left Chicago's city limits.

As I will describe in more depth in chapter 4, the immigration literature documents a paradox in immigrant health that is closely linked to the various forms of structural and interpersonal violence associated with migratory experiences. A growing body of research indicates that, while many immigrants come to Chicago in search of economic opportunity and a better life, they pay sometimes with steep social, psychological, and even physical costs—as demonstrated by the fact that the all-cause mortality of recent immigrants is significantly lower than the mortality rate of immigrant families who have lived in the United States for many years (Lara et al. 2005). Indeed, the health of the women in this book was severely compromised. My interlocutors' mental health was on average very poor: one in two women reported depression and 41 percent reported PTSD. The average body mass index was thirty-five, which is considered to be "extremely obese." Average blood pressure was 146/80, indicating that from a biomedical standpoint the typical study participant was "at risk" for further physical health complications (for example, being at risk for diabetes is set at 130/80). Most women in the study, in fact, had had diabetes for around a decade and reported at least two diabetes complications, indicating that their disease had progressed significantly. Further, all but nine of the women had poorly controlled diabetes.[15] Thus, the women interviewed for this book, living on the fringes of Mexican Chicago, may be understood to be extremely stressed and at considerable health risk. In many ways, they embody the broader health crisis of the inner-city poor in the United States (see Singer 1994).

Synthesizing VIDDA Syndemic Theory

The data explored in this book come from extensive mixed-methods interviews about stress, emotion, and diabetes collected during a ten-month period of fieldwork. I designed this study to combine qualitative and quantitative methods and made a point to place women's life stories at the center of my research. Like many medical anthropologists before me, I let the qualitative data shape my analysis, leaning on a grounded theory approach in which the categories analyzed were honed through evaluation of women's narratives. This approach is a distinctive departure from biomedical studies of stress and diabetes in which the investigator determines the course for analysis. My deductive technique is a more rigorous methodology when compared to evaluating life stressors through a general check-list, because the narratives provide in-depth description and contextualization that standardized surveys do not. This approach does not impose a priori assumptions or categories, but rather allows for the interlocutors to create meaning and define what matters in their lives.

My approach to conducting life history narrative interviews was largely open-ended. I intended to provide a space for women to speak freely about their life stories and, when necessary, gently guided them back to my research questions. I began each narrative interview with the simple question: "Can you tell me about your childhood?" Based on this question, and sometimes after more targeted probing such as "Where did you grow up?" and "Can you tell me about your family?" many women launched into detailed descriptions of their life stories. Additional questions included: "Have you ever been married?" "What age were you first married? Can you tell me about that relationship?" "Can you tell me about your family and your children?" "Have you ever experienced *coraje* (anger/rage)? If so, what caused it?" "Do any emotions affect your diabetes?" "What caused your diabetes?" "How do you manage your diabetes?" "Does anyone help you manage your diabetes?" and "Have you been depressed or hopeless in the last month?" Some women needed a great deal of prompting, but once broad questions were asked, and women began sharing their stories, the majority of them needed only limited inputs to address the themes at the heart of my study.

Many women spent much of the interview discussing extremely stressful aspects of their life stories. If a woman revealed minimal stress in her life narrative, I asked directly at the end of the interview if she had faced any traumatic or stressful experiences in her life. Because preliminary data indicated that interpersonal abuse was a major concern, I asked if my interlocutors had experienced any form of mistreatment or abuse if it was not previously mentioned. These prompts were given to only a handful of women, and the majority of them stated that they had not experienced interpersonal abuse or another form of severe stress. Thus, I concluded that most women reported distress without a great deal of direct probing.

Each interview was audiotaped and transcribed, and this body of text, together with my field notes, forms the core of my empirical material (the Spanish interviews have been translated into English for the purpose of this book). Text analysis often involves smaller datasets of twenty to thirty individuals, a number that is large enough to reach saturation of narrative themes but too small to evaluate the statistical associations of narrative themes with health outcomes (Bernard 1988). I reached saturation of narrative themes at around thirty interviews and could have crafted an informative qualitative analysis based on those data alone. However, I interviewed 121 women with the intent to use the narrative data differently than medical anthropologists typically do. In addition to analyzing the common themes emanating from women's stories, I quantified major life stresses and put these data into regression analyses of health outcomes. This approach enabled me to determine how stress in women's lives might interact with the clustering of depression with diabetes in this population, a central tenet of VIDDA Syndemic theory.

I conducted narrative analysis in two stages, roughly corresponding to the open coding and axial coding approaches used in grounded theory (Strauss and Corbin 1990). For open coding, I analyzed my field notes in order to generate narrative themes, including "abuse," "health stress," "family stress," and "social stress." Then, I used axial coding to identify any mention of these narrative themes across the transcripts and scrutinize the variations within these larger themes (Bernard 1988). I used both field notes and transcripts to ensure that any mention of these themes was recorded into the database that was prepared for quantitative analyses.

It was the process of evaluating the many layers of qualitative data alone and together with markers of mental and physical health that fueled my understanding of the VIDDA Syndemic. First, by examining women's life history narratives I was able to observe the trajectory of stress throughout the life course and understand how such stress may have interacted with or perpetuated other forms of acutely traumatic experience. Second, I scoured women's stories and systematically recorded the main forms of chronic stress and acute distress that women carried with them as defining moments in their lives. These major stresses, described in depth in chapter 3, include a history of interpersonal abuse, feelings of social isolation, the stress associated with health, immigration, and work, the loss of a family member, family discord, financial difficulties, and neighborhood violence. Finally, I took the most commonly reported life stresses and evaluated their association with measures of depression and post-traumatic stress disorder (PTSD).

Thus, VIDDA Syndemic theory emerged organically through a ground-up, evidence-based methodology. My systematic, multistep analysis of mixed qualitative and quantitative data provides a narrative perspective of the social factors that are at the root of increasing rates of depression, diabetes, and their overlap and entwinement among low-income Mexican immigrant women in Chicago. By critically examining their stories and systematically evaluating individual and common trends, this book reveals the rich content of my interlocutors' lives and the intimate connections between *V*iolence, *I*mmigration, *D*epression, *D*iabetes, and *A*buse.

2

SYNERGIES OF THE SELF:
THE ENDURANCE OF SYNDEMIC SUFFERING

In 1961, John L. Austin's lectures on *How to Do Things with Words* revolution-ized the way in which people thought about words, and texts more generally. Austin challenged literary scholars to move beyond the belief that an utterance functioned solely as a communicative statement that could be either true or false. Utterances are not just to "say" something; rather, such statements provide rich information that moves beyond the texts themselves to perform a certain kind of action, such as making a point, sparking emotion, or influencing behavior. Since then, literary scholars have interpreted people's "speech acts" not as mere texts, but as performative acts through which individuals construct meaning and define their "self" in the world (Bauman 1986; Bruner 1986; Atkinson 1990; Reissman 1990; Mattingly 1998).

Researchers have found in the examination of illness narratives a unique opportunity for understanding how patients conceptualize causes of and experi-ences with disease. They have found that patients use these narratives not only to explain their suffering to others, but also to make sense of the illness experience for themselves. Through illness narration, individuals struggle to bridge their past, present, future, and even imagined lives to formulate coherent identities (Bruner 1986; Capps and Ochs 1995; Mattingly 1998; Garro and Mattingly 2000).

A chronic illness such as diabetes transforms and disrupts the everyday lived experience of people who suffer from it. As such, tales about living with a chronic illness and making sense of its causes are central to diabetes narratives.

These narratives may function as tools with which patients actively refigure a "self" that has been severely undermined by the illness experience (Ochs and Capps 1996; Becker 1997; Hunt 1998; Mattingly 1998; Hunt 2000). In this sense, narratives have a therapeutic dimension when patients use them to reconcile expectation with experience (Labov 1972; Kleinman 1980; Kleinman 1988; Pennebaker 1997; Mattingly 1998; Seligman 2005).

In addition, some scholars have argued that patients use narrative strategically to influence their social situations (Hunt 1998, 2000; Mattingly 1998). Linda M. Hunt (2000) found that Mexican cancer patients built causal stories about their illnesses based on local moral constructs framed within distinct cultural and social perspectives. These cancer patients strove to make their illnesses meaningful in terms of everyday life, and strategically reconfigured their identities in ways that were socially empowering. For example, a wife who dealt with thirty years of domestic abuse cited her husband's abuse as the cause of her brain cancer, publicly challenging him and being recognized as his victim for the first time. Literature on domestic violence finds that victims of physical and sexual abuse hesitate to tell their stories and when they do, their stories often have a fragmented character (Herman 1992; Polletta 2007). However, Hunt demonstrates that finding a way to talk about abuse can function as a source of empowerment. The patients in Hunt's study effected change at the microsocial level without challenging or overtly protesting larger political-economic forces. At the same time, their narratives articulate their relationship to these larger macrosocial forces by illustrating how such forces affect their lived experience.

Individuals may also use illness narratives to identify distressing experiences from their pasts that continue to affect their everyday lives and consequently may interact with the management and treatment of the chronic illness itself. Because the lives of people with chronic illnesses have already been disrupted by the disease, they may strategically use their affliction to make sense of, and reorder, elements of their biographies that continue to live on through powerful memories. As such, the revision of the self-narrative becomes part of the chronic illness, as in reconstructing their memory of the life they have lived people may prioritize the experiences that were similarly difficult or linked with their newly diseased self. Therefore, "strategic suffering" is both a social tool for reconfiguring identity and a tool for making sense of ongoing stress and psychological anguish.

In the next pages I introduce two life stories to demonstrate how individuals use narratives to make sense of their suffering and their condition, and why narratives are useful tools for developing syndemics theory. These two cases reveal some of the most extreme forms of social distress reported by the women in my study and illustrate the complicated interface of social, psychological, and physical distress that is a corollary of the VIDDA Syndemic.

Domenga's Story

Domenga is a 51-year-old mother of three who was born in Jalisco, Mexico. She moved to the United States at thirteen years of age, but returned to Mexico after one year to care for her siblings. She re-emigrated to Chicago at the age of twenty, and currently lives in Pilsen, a predominantly Mexican immigrant neighborhood. We met in the General Medicine Clinic and spent around six hours together, including both informal and formal interviewing.

"I am from Mexico, from the state of Jalisco," Domenga began as she eased herself into the booth at the far end of the cafeteria. Hot soup sat in front her as she leaned forward to speak clearly into the audio recorder. Seemingly uninterested in her lunch, Domenga continued,

> I come from a rural area, and we moved to a small city that was located near Guadalajara, the capital of the state, when I was ten years old. Then, when I was thirteen my parents took me to Chicago. The first time I came here, I was thirteen and we stayed here for about a year. Then, I moved back to Jalisco for four to five years [to take care of my siblings]. My mother, younger sister born in Chicago, and father stayed. We stayed alone in Mexico and took care of each other.

Domenga sat up straight on the other side of the booth with her hands crossed in front of her on the table. She spoke directly and carefully into the audio recorder, like she was proud to tell her story and aware that someone would be listening. When not looking at the recorder, Domenga's eyes darted around the cafeteria and sometimes locked with mine as she spoke.

> We didn't have enough money to eat, so I began working, and my siblings too. We cleaned houses, worked in supermarkets, and worked in little stores in the neighborhood. After work, we would sometimes spend time with our grand parents [. . .] I didn't study, but I learned bookkeeping. I worked as a cashier in a discotheque. It was a lot of work when we were young, but we had the strength, and we were able to do many things.
>
> Eventually we decided to go to the U.S. [when I was 20 years old], because it was too much suffering for the family to be apart. We passed through Tijuana, over the hills, with coyotes. We had to pay them $500 each for us to pass. It was me, my sister, my brother. This included money for the trip, [guidance to travel] over the hills/path, to take us to a house for a few days and give us food to eat for the trip, and a plane ticket. The mosquitoes bit us at night, and we were all very young, but protected. The helicopters didn't see us during our trip because they are all very high, and the area is very arid, very dry. There are mountains that we had to climb up and down, and we resembled the landscape, we escaped among the vegetation. In some way we passed at night there and we were able to pass. We arrived in Los

Angeles, and then went to Chicago where our father picked us up. And that is another story altogether that includes many things, many bad stories that include my father.

I was about twenty [when we arrived back in Chicago to live]. It's hard for me to talk about [that time], because I have shame. I didn't know what [my father] was thinking and didn't believe what was happening. All I knew was that I had to get out of my father's house. He wouldn't let me go to the movies, I couldn't leave my house for anything, I couldn't have friends. We lived on the fourth floor, and he wouldn't let me down [. . .] If I'd return five minutes late from work [in a factory] he would hit me in the face, and other things happened that were even more horrible. But I can't talk about them without shaking and crying. It's true that I am stronger, and that my history is very long, like I said.

Like many women I met, Domenga initially spoke of her father's abuse in passing. She mentioned that traumatic memories from her childhood were still affecting her, and psychiatric inventories indicated that she had symptoms of PTSD (PCL-C: 32) and severe depression (CES-D: 30).[1] I asked Domenga if she had been abused and she responded that her father raped her when she immigrated to the United States at twenty years of age. Although very few women felt comfortable sharing with me the intimate details of past abuse, Domenga had spoken openly about difficult situations. I asked her if she would be interested in talking more in depth about what happened and if I could turn the audio recorder back on. She agreed and spoke for an additional thirty minutes.

I had to go to a shelter because one day he [my father] wanted to abuse me, to hit me in the face, and I knew I had to take control of the situation. I thought, he is going to throw me across the room. I said, "This is a small place, the door is there, and someone will hear me, and I can call someone." But the telephone was in the other room, and I didn't realize that the door was closed and I was locked in. It was almost ten in the night, and everyone was sleeping. I was in my pajamas and socks. When I realized it, I asked, "Why is the door closed?" He said to come here. No more than to come here. He said that he just wanted to sleep with me for awhile. I thought, sleep with me, why?

But then I quickly realized, it had come up in my mind the other times, not just then, but other times when he had insinuated things, and when he said, because he had another time, when he suggested he go to bed with me. I had said, no no no. He was crazy, and had forgotten that I was his daughter, and he wanted to be with me. What did he want to do? And when I realized his intentions, I began to scream. Nobody heard me in the building. A building on the fourth floor, with many people. Nobody heard me scream, and scream. Don't do this to me. Don't you know that I'm your daughter? The thoughts came quickly to me; that I just had to have the strength to get through this reality. At that time I didn't think of my little sister. He began to hit me on the face, in the head, in the mouth, he began beating me. Eventually, when I reacted, he didn't understand. He said that there was a demon in there. I wanted to find strength and close my legs so he would stop. [*The description becomes very graphic and is omitted*]

I escaped and went running down the stairs to the third, then the second, floor. I ran to my comadre [aunt/Godmother], and I cried and cried. I said that my father beat me, and I had blood on my face. They said that they would call the police, and I hid in the closet. I asked them not to call the police, because I was thinking what I would say to them [. . .] I was still waiting for my papers, it is a process of legalization and is something that we had to prepare for my mother and siblings. I knew they would put charges toward my father and put him in jail, and he could not take care of my mother and siblings. My little sister is the only person I cared about, and I thought of her [. . .] I later discovered that my younger sister suffered from my father's abuse for five years.

— physical abuse
— sexual abuse
— hopless
— scared
— situational obligations

Domenga eventually gained citizenship, but this did not shield her from the chronically severe stresses of everyday life that are common among the poor and the working class in the United States. A decade after the abuse, Domenga went through another traumatic experience that had profound social and economic repercussions in her life story. She had met and married a Mexican man who "came from the same town, and came [to Chicago] the same year, to the same neighborhood." Although they did not know each other initially, her brother introduced them and they eventually married. But by the age of thirty-one Domenga was on her own again with two young girls:

My husband was killed in an accident in 1989. [He worked for] a demolition company. He fell 150 feet up, at work. He was with another guy. They were cutting a bridge that was holding a building. An African American and him—they both were killed. And it's been twenty years, but it's still hard. It's been very difficult. It's just the way life is. You never forget. You just accept the reality.

— death — no grieving?

Initially, Domenga swallowed her sorrow and cared for her two young children, financially and emotionally, rarely providing space for herself to grieve. She explained:

[I dealt with it through my] faith in God. I just think that I'm not the only one. I'm not the only one who has faced these situations. There are other people in this world who have lost more than me. I was asking God, why me, why me? Then, a voice told me, why are you a coward? Why do you ask so much? You are not special in this world. There are more people who suffer more than you, and lose more relatives. You just have to ask God to be strong, and keep going. To do your best taking care of your children. To educate my daughters in the best way possible. Taking them to places and different activities to keep them out of gangs, drugs, bullies, who are in the schools.

faith — protective factor.
changed behavior/ outlook for siblings/ kids

You know, my daughters maybe are not the best. They may not do the best as others. But they finish their schools: grammar schools, secondary schools, and college. With the exception of my daughter who was in the university when she got sick [with bipolar disorder]. But she's like me. She's always trying to go back and finish. Always go back. Everyday, you try again. You fall, and you pick yourself up again. It's the way life is. Did you ever see the pink panther? It's like the pink panther. You know, she got run over by a car, and was stuck to the road like a sticker. She picked up her luggages and went on in life again. That's what we're supposed to be.

DMDx:
"luggage"

When Domenga was later diagnosed with diabetes, she similarly applied the trope of "going on with life again." While some women reported that initially the diagnosis was somewhat traumatizing, many seemed to have accepted, or simply ignored, their disease as time went on. In a sense, diabetes became one of the many stresses a woman packed into her "luggages." I asked Domenga how she found out that she was diabetic, and she explained:

> I found out [that I had diabetes] because I was taking some classes when I was thirty-five years old and I started losing my vision. My vision was really blurry. Sometimes I wasn't eating breakfast, and I was feeling really tired. I was feeling tingling in my hands, like someone was pinching my fingers and toes. My mouth was really dry. I was thirsty and feeling really weak. I was thirty-five and by that time I was experiencing a lot of pressure. When my husband was killed, I was in shock. Probably I had symptoms before, but I never realized it. That's when I started going to the doctor, but I didn't go too often [. . .].
>
> Initially I was depressed. I stopped taking the medicine for a year and it made me forget many things, and when I started taking the medicines again a year later, it had affected me so much. I don't know if it's the medicine or all that has happened to me, but I have forgotten many doctor appointments, forgetting many things, and then I just forget my medicines. [pause] I am able to control my disease well, passing through normal phases of depression, sadness, and more or less calm.

takes care
of others
before
themselves:

Near the end of ninety minutes of dialogue, Domenga's soup was cold, but she didn't seem to mind. She had waved off my numerous suggestions that we take a break and eat, saying that she enjoyed our conversation too much to eat. She repeated that rarely could she speak so freely about her life experiences, let alone have time to focus on herself. In fact, Domenga repeated throughout our conversation that she often prioritized her families' needs before her own, even in relation to diabetes self-care:

> I didn't take good care of myself because I had so many people to care for: my mother, my younger sister, my daughters, my grandson. There wasn't time to take responsibility for myself and I wasn't feeling bad all of the time. When I did feel bad, I'd tell myself that I wasn't doing 100 percent for my people, my loved ones,

myself. I wasn't taking care of myself. I wasn't taking a shower every day. I was starting to look very depressed. I was so depressed and had so much anxiety. I wanted to cry all the time.

When I was depressed in the past, I didn't take medicines. Now I take Zoloft, at first 25 mg and then 50. And now I am taking it, and slowly I am forgetting things and I am realizing that I really need it. When I was experiencing a really strong depression, I felt it in my entire organism and I couldn't do anything. I was very sad. My sugar levels were extremely high also, up to four hundred before lunch. And it was horrifying to eat because I [pause] It might have given me an attack again, right?

Domenga's story mirrored others I found in my study, characterized by fluid interactions between the feelings associated with past abuse, ongoing emotional strife, and diabetes. Additionally, women often discussed diabetes as a manifestation of age and multiple experiences of distress, as a consequence of a hard life. Domenga continued:

When I didn't have diabetes, I was a very active person. I was not sad. All day long I was going, all day long. I would say hyperactive because I always wanted to be doing something. And now I don't have the same level of activity. I move like a robot, slowly. I am often confused, and I forget a lot of things, many things and I forget doctor appointments. It's a combination of age and diabetes, and everything. It could be also a combination of what's going on with my menopause, and the diabetes affects my mind a great deal. I have read that it affects my sight and hearing too, and also my nervous system because my blood doesn't have the components that it needs, the sugar. The blood is not pure because our pancreas, and all that, fails to produce the pure blood. Thus, it affects our kidneys and all the organs in our body, and as a result affects how our nervous system works, our principle organs and our physical body. Because of this, I feel very sad, very weak, and without a lot of energy to do things [. . .].

Many people take drastic measures and become too depressed, and think that their ignorance caused their diabetes, and other people become completely incapacitated. They can't do anything, they become completely depressed, and begin to affect their symptoms.

Domenga began to move in her seat. We were near the end of the interview and I could sense that she was beginning to move beyond the topic of diabetes. She concluded: "I'm sad to say that all of this happened. If there is one day you want me to, then I can tell you everything, everything, everything. Yes, like I said, my life is like a novel that is not yet complete."

As I listened to Domenga's words, and later in reviewing the transcript, this statement stuck with me and made me think about the narrative process through which Domenga crafted her life story. In *Actual Minds, Possible Worlds* Jerome Bruner states, "What is 'given' or assumed at the onset of our construction [of narrative] is neither bedrock reality out there, nor an a priori: it is always another constructed version of a world that we have taken as given for certain purposes" (1986, 97). Many scholars embrace this notion of subjectivity and argue that storytelling is a process through which individuals make sense of past experience and produce a notion of "the self" that is dependent on time and context (Labov 1972; Bruner 1986; Kirby 1991; Freeman 1993; McAdams 1996; Ochs and Capps 1996; Langellier 2001). Domenga's narrative must be understood as closely interconnected with her current understanding of her self and the particular self she wished, or perhaps *needed*, to present in her interaction with me, a stranger who was not linked with her social network but was associated with the trusted institution from which she received diabetes care. Now a late-adult woman with diabetes, Domenga uses her narrative to construct a resilient self that continues to pack the stresses of everyday life into her luggage and go on with life again.

Rosie's Story

Rosie is a 59-year-old woman who never married or had children of her own, and invested much of her life in working for Chicago Public Schools. Rosie lost her job due to what she calls "race politics" after holding a high-level administrative position for more than ten years. Because her health had deteriorated over the past several years, and her insurance had failed to cover many of her expenses, Rosie decided to accept a large severance in lieu of a stable pension for public service so that she could pay off her substantial medical debt. Five years later Rosie remained unemployed; she had lost her home, was living on a friend's couch, and was seeking medical care for psychiatric and physical problems at Cook County's General Medicine Clinic.

In a private room adjacent to the GMC, Rosie explained that the root of her psychological suffering was a traumatic experience from childhood. She sat stoically during much of our dialogue, carefully choosing her words and speaking to me as a teacher instructs a student. Solemnly but matter-of-factly, she explained that she was kidnapped and raped by a stranger at the age of seven. Even though the media covered this event extensively, her family never spoke of it, and as an adult she educated herself about the event through Chicago's media channels. She stated, "I know only from the newspaper that I was [kidnapped]—he kept me for about three days and then he left me on a road [pause] and someone picked me up and brung [*sic*] me to the town." When I asked her, "Do you ever talk about what happened to you?" she replied, "Never." I continued with, "Do your friends know?" She replied, "No. Only my psychiatrist [knows], who's in this hospital [and I've be been seeing him for] three years now." Rosie only began meeting with the psychiatrist two years after seeking health services in the Cook County system, which was also when she was diagnosed with diabetes. She had never sought mental health care through her private insurance due to the cost.

I asked her if the abuse from more than fifty years ago still affected her life. Rosie replied,

> Yeah, it affects your attention span at times. Although by the time that I decided to seek—to talk about it with a psychiatrist, my life was already complete in terms of education, number of years on the job [pause] and all of that. But throughout my life, no, this would be the second time [that I talk about it].

I probed, "Did you ever have dreams about it?"

> Well, I—I still have dreams about it. Like once I started speaking with my—with Dr. Smith [*pseudonym*], who's the psychiatrist here. Then, I have somewhat of flashbacks in my dreams where he puts his hand on my mouth, and I'm trying to yell and yell. And I couldn't, you know, and I do this kind of movement [crosses arms and moves abruptly from side to side]. But I've never seen his face. I only see his hand. So, yes, it's troubling. That's why I have sleeping pills, and I truly believe that my anxiety disorders come from that incident. It is totally linked to it.

When I asked if the early childhood abuse was linked with diabetes, too, Rosie replied:

> Well, diabetes is a totally different world that—if it's a link it has to do with depression. When I developed depression, I was in my teens, as a result of the rape. [pause] The kidnap and the rape. Now I have diabetes. My depression is more consistent than when I was in my teens because I have to think about: are they going to amputate my leg? Am I going to go blind? I mean, and that, for me as a person, causes me to be depressed. And then, the lack of resources. [pause] Because I lost my home [. . .].
>
> I was the only Hispanic who had reached the level of deputy superintendent [in my school district]. Then, the management changed, and I knew that when the management would change, that I would be out because they would want to put their own. The town was 99 percent Hispanic but everyone [who worked at the school] there are from Poland. They're Americans, of course. They don't live in the community [but] they work there. At the time that happened, I was fifty-five. Then I got sick. I was diagnosed with diabetes. I was diagnosed with anxiety disorders, and I have panic attacks from time to time. Less, less, and less every month, but . . .

I was intrigued by Rosie's thoughtful interpretation of her life story. In her opinion, her anxiety and panic were related to what had happened to her as a

[margin handwriting: economic insuuity, lack of institutional support]

young person, but her depression was linked to diabetes. Rosie emphasized the pivotal influence of economic insecurity and lack of institutional support on her health condition, and went on to discuss these interactions in greater detail when we discussed her diabetes onset:

> Well, diabetes is hereditary. I truly believe at that time I would eat anything at any time. [I was] stressed-out. I worked sixty to seventy hours a week. I was responsible for fifteen schools: not one school—fifteen schools. So my stress level was very, very high and I compensated by eating whatever I wanted at any time I wanted. So, the factors to get diabetes are family, stress, and bad eating habits. [pause] Very bad eating habits.

I was interested in Rosie's perceptions of the interconnectedness of these symptoms and health problems, so I asked if she thought that the depression was linked with what happened to her and if her being depressed for such a long period of time had influenced her diabetes. She stated:

[margin handwriting: loss of resources —sense of helplessness to lose all resources]

> It made it worse. No, no, oh no, I think that [pause] when a person suffers from depression like me [pause] okay, and I managed it the best I could so I could, you know, go to work, graduate from college, and so on and so forth, [it] makes the disease seem much bigger. [pause] Overwhelming. [. . .] Well, it seems overwhelming because now if we look at the incident, right, it happened when I was seven years old. However, there were—I truly believe that at that time I experienced stressors as a child that sort of marked the amount of worry in my life. So now I have diabetes, and diabetes goes into all aspects of one's life.
>
> So therefore, it's like I have a cape, not to protect myself, but a cape to remind me, that I have to do sugar, that I have to eat certain foods. [pause] I mean, everything becomes very aggravated because I don't have the resources that I [pause] I mean, I made $100,000 before, and now I receive $670 per month from Social Security, so in the process I lost my home. [pause] I owned my home. Now I live at my friend's [place], you know, [she] rent[s] me a room [. . .]. I have tried [to get another job], but now I'm disabled, because [*crying*] No, no, it's okay. I have to—if you give me a second. [*Rosie began to cry as I handed her a tissue and gave her time to settle down.*]
> Because I have anxiety disorders and panic attacks. I have glaucoma, I have dead bladder. I have bladder neuropathy; it doesn't function. That's when I said, the money that you're contributing to me is going to go to buy catheters. Because this clinic—this hospital is unable to buy catheters and the cheapest catheter is 98 cents per catheter. So you see how the impact, everything is linked. I truly believe that at age five if a child is put [under] some stressors, like being taken and going through the rape in a span of three days. [pause] Three days, as a child, you don't know if it's

long or short or whatever. But it's a different world because they took me from a nurturing—he took me from a nurturing environment to the pits of hell.

During our conversation Rosie sat straight as an arrow across the table from me. For much of the time she kept her hands carefully folded on the table. When I first met her, there was no indication that she was distressed, as opposed to some women who appeared downtrodden or fidgety. However, Rosie's score for PTSD on the PCL-C was 63, which is an extremely high score, and the symptomatology from the PCL-C indicated that she had recurrent nightmares revisiting the traumatic event of her childhood and she maintained hypervigilance in her environment because she was always on edge and aware of potential threats. Rosie articulated clearly how the feelings linked with early childhood trauma continued to affect her:

PTSD - on edge / potential threat - surveys environment

> I think to lessen some of the degrees of anxiety, and somewhat depression, I would need safety. Because I've never felt in my life that I was safe. I'm a grown person and still, because that incident occur[ed], that I was taken. It's not that I'm just hiding, that I don't go out or anything like that. It's just that it's so marked in my emotional well-being, and you know, in my emotional make-up rather, it's that that is something a person lives with. I cannot leave it behind. Like I don't—cannot leave behind my arm here and go home. It's just constantly with me. [pause] And with many people that were raped [pause] I cannot speak about the rape or anything like that, but as a child, it's just like another big book that you are taking to school [. . .].
>
> Well, the good thing [is that flashbacks] happen when I am sleeping. It has to do with my sleeping patterns, and the medication that I'm on now has really helped. I don't wake up at one or two o'clock just to wander around in my room or whatever. No, so it has really helped. And also Dr. Smith is a very good provider.

I asked her if she felt safe with him.

> Yeah, yeah. Well, what I mean [by] safety is, for example, I don't know anything about your life and I'm not pretending to know anything about your life either, but let's say a person, who didn't—who was never raped or kidnapped—because rape is one thing, kidnap is another. In the emotional state of a five-year-old, it's not that I'm a five-year-old, I know very well my age and where I'm at, and what I need to manage, and I manage. [pause] It's that on a daily basis there are reminders that I was raped, and then the safety issue comes to [pause] would I be raped again?

At the same time Rosie reported symptoms of severe depression (CES-D: 29). I asked Rosie if emotion affected her diabetes, and she explained:

severe depression

> Well it affects more my depression, and then, as a consequence, then diabetes is something I have to put [pause] It's a focus of my life because if I control the, you

know, if I manage well my diet and medicines, and so on, well, I feel better so the depression is going to go down. But if I'm very, very depressed, I don't want to get up or whatever, then diabetes suffers. Symptoms of diabetes will become more complicated. Because when, I don't know if you have ever been depressed, but the correction is unique to the person, it's unique to the person's experiences or lack of experiences. So if I'm very, very depressed, I want to make sure to take my depression medication so I can then prepare my foods, you know, personal hygiene, and so on and so forth. So I can be much more aware to manage the glucose. See? So it's complicated.

I asked Rosie how diabetes had affected her life. "Well I think in positive ways," she replied, "because if I was not diagnosed with diabetes I wouldn't—I would still have a very poor diet. And when I started this program, I was 217 pounds, and now I am 184, so gradually, I have been able to do some good things. Or create new habits so that I can manage." When I asked if diabetes affected her feelings, she went on to explain,

> No. Not any more. In the beginning, yes. It was like, because it's a chronic disease. So if you think about diabetes as being the illness that can be managed, self-management, [then] it's something to cope with. It's easier to cope with. But if I think [about] diabetes as a chronic disease who will impact my life, I could go blind, renal failure, amputation, and so on and so forth, that is a different level, it's a higher lever of stress.

I probed, "So your diabetes is well controlled today?" She replied bluntly, "I have managed, with my resources, the best I can."

Synergies of the Self

These two stories clearly illuminate how *V*iolence, *I*mmigration, *D*epression, *D*iabetes, and *A*buse are synergistically interconnected. First, structural violence played a central role in each woman's story, through lack of institutional support, and specifically the lack of social protection evident in Domenga's story. Second, both women felt socially isolated in some way: Domenga felt as though she was the thread holding her family together while no one was caring for her needs, and Rosie had very few people in her life to support her and largely coped alone. Indeed, this second point must be situated within the larger framework of immigration and the related transitions and transformations of the social fabric of families. Third, both women described feeling extreme psychiatric distress, in the form of symptoms of depression, anxiety, and PTSD linked with past traumatic experience and ongoing chronic disease. Fourth, diabetes was a stressor that had affected both women's lives; however, neither woman placed diabetes at the center of her story. Importantly, diabetes was one of many stresses in their lives, and women gave the disease less weight than other stresses (such as family discord or depression). Finally, experiences of sexual abuse during adolescence and early adulthood were extremely powerful memories for both women. These experiences were kept private and largely internalized for many years before they were openly identified as a major contributor to psychiatric distress. Combined, these five key factors make up the VIDDA Syndemic and clearly contributed to the extreme suffering in Domenga's and Rosie's lives.

Stories like Domenga's and Rosie's should be situated in a larger political context that associates increasing wealth disparities and lack of social welfare with a rise in violence against women (Goode and Maskovsky 2001; Wilkinson and Pickett 2009). David Harvey has argued, "The loss of social protections in advanced capitalist countries has had particularly negative effects on lower-class women" (2005, 170). This loss of social protection is exemplified by Domenga's story of abuse and provides the most acute illustration of how macrolevel phenomena become realized in individual experience. During the aggression Domenga recalls calling for help and receiving no response in the close-quartered apartment building. After the incident, Domenga did not seek legal protection from her father due to her undocumented status, and her lack of English proficiency prevented her from seeking alternate services. Moreover, Domenga understood her father to be the family breadwinner and would not risk jeopardizing the economic stability of her family by prosecuting him. In this sense, social welfare and legal services (the "state") failed to protect her from sexual abuse and its repercussions. Thus, Domenga experienced a perfect storm of victimization: she felt powerless and vulnerable in the private and political spheres, fearing both her father's wrath and the political and legal problems that would develop if she reported the abuse.

Indeed, various forms of structural, symbolic, and gender-based violence are clearly at work in Domenga's life story. Structural violence plays a central role as a major contributor to her family's economic needs and determination to relocate to Chicago, thereby breaking up the family for many years. Symbolic violence figures in Domenga's fear and shame to talk to others about her father's transgression; and shame also possibly contributed in some way to her father's violent acts toward his daughter. In other words, the inexcusable violence he laid upon his daughter might have stemmed from some sense of insecurity and from the desire to reaffirm the power that he had lost in the public sphere.

Rosie's story incorporates similar experiences—such as the structural limitations associated with the loss of her job, the racial discrimination she perceived as the force behind the loss of her career, and the gendered violence she recounted as a major cause of her ongoing emotional distress. In addition, Rosie explained that her soaring medical bills put her in a poor position to maintain her level of financial security, forcing her into a low-income status that made her dependent on the health care safety net. However, Rosie's story is a unique case, not only because of the extreme act of violence she experienced as a young person, but also because she was fairly well-off financially for much of her adult life and had access to health insurance. According to her life story, only when her health deteriorated did things begin to unravel. Nevertheless, Rosie's story shows how precarious immigrant women's economic status can be: even though Rosie achieved economic security, her structural vulnerability forced her into relative poverty once her job unraveled and medical bills soared, thereby pushing her to join the status of other lower-income women.

Indeed, Rosie's diabetes diagnosis seemed to represent a pivotal shift in her life story. Unlike Domenga's story, which seemed to follow a somewhat chronological narrative arc, Rosie sharply jumped from her childhood trauma to her struggles with diabetes decades later. This explains her "struggle to achieve coherence and continuity rather than objective truth" (Capps and Ochs 1995, 15); in other words, Rosie sought to find continuity and give order and meaning to her chaotic past by emphasizing the emotional interconnections between childhood trauma and diabetes. It may be that in fact diabetes made Rosie begin to confront the traumatic memories of her past, since her present suffering awoke raw memories that she had tried to bury for years. Therefore, the diabetes diagnosis held significant value for her as a way to make sense of the legacy of childhood trauma on her life story and as a constant irritant that contributed to other forms of misery, such as the loss of a past successful life. In this way, Rosie's diabetes made her even more vulnerable to being depressed and reliving her past traumatic experience.

Laurence Kirmayer (1992) has argued that two orders affect people's experiences with illness: the order of the body, and the order of the text (or narrative). As Rosie's story demonstrates, an inescapable circularity exists between the two: when people are unable to make sense of the disorder of the body, narrative functions as a process of reconciliation through which they work through changing understandings of their emotional, social, and diseased self. Gay Becker opines, "When the body is assaulted by a serious illness, one's sense of wholeness, on which a sense of order rides, disintegrates. One must constitute that sense of wholeness in order to regain a sense of continuity" (1997, 39). Soon after Rosie was diagnosed with diabetes she began to see a psychiatrist and, for the first time, addressed her emotional needs. When Rosie shared her story with me, five years after being diagnosed with diabetes, she largely glossed over nearly forty years of her life between the traumatic experience and the diagnosis, probably because she had learned to create some sort of coherence in her life story through connecting these two significant events. Perhaps if she were interviewed ten years before, she might not have woven the trauma from early childhood into her life story. But these two stressful events became central to her current sense of self, even though these two stressful experiences bookended many years of relative success. By interweaving these seemingly disparate events, then, Rosie was able to inscribe some sense of order into a disordered past. She made visible the "mark" of childhood trauma in her physical problems and identified such traumatic experience as corollary to both her psychiatric and metabolic conditions, recognizing the coherence of trauma and diabetes that fueled her emotional devastation.

Finally, Rosie's story introduces an interesting point I will return to throughout this book: following the diabetes diagnosis, Rosie began to seek mental health care for her mental anguish. It is not surprising that many women in my study, particularly those who were undocumented or Spanish-speaking, would delay seeking diabetes care and at the same time fail to seek institutional support for their psychological distress. However, Rosie was an exception: she had private health insurance through her high-level administrative position and could have visited a psychiatrist long before the onset of diabetes. Rosie, as did many women, only came to address her psychological distress through her institutional access to the safety net of the hospital system, and through her diabetes care began to see that she needed to tend to the mind to tend to the body. In addition, the emotions she associated with diabetes might have brought to light other emotional experiences, increasing her need for mental health care. In other words, the emotions associated with diabetes might have been too overwhelming to deal with on top of the other experiences from which she still suffered. As such, her diabetes diagnosis functioned as an access point and a turning moment to address her mental and physical health.

While this seemed to be true for some other study participants, there were also institutional barriers associated with mental health care that prevented many women from receiving the services they needed. Indeed, both narratives provide evidence of how poor access to mental health care—Rosie by putting it off, and Domenga by medicating the problem rather than receiving opportunities for talk therapy—may contribute to prolonged emotional problems that, in turn, might contribute to risk factors for chronic disease and may later interact with the disease itself. Indeed, I found that Spanish-speaking women like Domenga[2] rarely had access to mental health care, and when they did, they often felt dismissed by clinicians.

However, the language barrier was not always the cause of such limited access. An English-speaking respondent stated, "I haven't seen a psychiatrist now because there's a waiting list. But I am taking an antidepressant." Certainly, the use of medication in lieu of (instead of in tandem with) talk therapy should not be attributed solely to the fact that these women sought care from a safety-net clinic. This is a far greater national challenge for mental health care in the United States: most insurance companies would rather pay for medication as opposed to talk therapy. Indeed, the number of women who reported receiving an antidepressant prescription indicates that the mental anguish of these women had been acknowledged by their physicians in some capacity—regardless of the fact that the physicians might or might not have acknowledged, or fully understood, the roots of their psychological suffering.

Even more, diabetes compliance might be the main goal of many physicians who prescribe antidepressants for people with poor diabetes control. When physicians at the GMC believe that a patient may be experiencing some psychiatric distress, they make an appointment with the psychiatrist for a prescription. However, because of the institutional barriers that do not allow these women to receive psychotherapy, it is unlikely that their psychological needs are met. Even the best physicians at the GMC acknowledged that they rarely considered the role of domestic abuse in diabetes care.

Conclusion

Narratives function as unique windows into the lives of individuals with chronic illness. Without narrative-level analysis it would be easy to dismiss the women in this study simply as *victims* of VIDDA Syndemic interactions. In a sense, they might become another statistic. However, it is not my intent to portray Domenga or Rosie as victims. Both intense suffering and incredible resilience seep through Domenga's and Rosie's stories, and their life narratives reveal, as Lancaster puts it, the *"endurance* of the people who survive life's hardships" (1994, xvi; italics in the original).

Even more, the stories show how important it is to understand the interconnections of structural, social, interpersonal, psychological, and metabolic factors that contribute to the health and well-being of the women in my sample at large. Understanding such synergies require in-depth study and creative interventions that move beyond the simple band-aid approaches commonly provided in safety-net care networks. However, simply focusing on women's stories without systematically evaluating the syndemic interactions of social and emotional factors with psychological and biological ones remains limited in that it does not show specific ways in which narrative accounts might communicate actual diseases. The next chapter, therefore, moves beyond narrative analysis and uses grounded theory to systematically catalogue the major forms of chronic stress and acute distress reported across the dataset. These narrative themes are explained in depth, setting up for their application in the regression analyses presented in chapter 5.

3

UNPACKING VIDDA:
AN ANALYSIS OF SOCIAL STRESS

Before I started collecting the narratives for this study I projected that diabetes would be one, if not *the* principal, stressor in the lives of the women I met. This hypothesis was based primarily on diabetes scholarship, which has documented a large number of undiagnosed people with diabetes in the general population (Cowie et al. 2010), and on health services research, which has found Latinos to be more likely to delay care-seeking than other ethnic groups in the United States due to issues of documentation, racism, and other access barriers (de la Torre et al. 1996; Amaro and de la Torre 2002). As a result, I predicted that my interlocutors would have advanced diabetes symptoms, such as loss of eyesight and other troubling side effects, and that therefore diabetes problems would be at the center of their narratives. Indeed, the women I met were not just living with chronic illness. Most of them had had diabetes and other chronic diseases for more than a decade.

Early in my research I discovered that the women I interviewed put much lower priority on their diabetes than I did. This was despite the fact that, as suspected, more than 90 percent of my interlocutors had poorly controlled diabetes (HbA1c ≥ 6.5), the average number of diabetes complications was slightly more than two, and severe complications were not uncommon. Many women had advanced microvascular problems, such as kidney failure, loss of eyesight, and numbing in the extremities due to nerve damage; yet these complications represented only a fraction of the stress communicated in their life histories. I do not mean to diminish the impact of diabetes in people's lives; many women identified their chronic illness to be a major source of chronic stress. Rather, I mean to communicate that in a group in which most had poorly controlled diabetes, it was alarming to realize the severity and centrality of stress factors apart from diabetes.

In this chapter I first situate these findings into a broader discussion about stress and diabetes among Mexican and Mexican immigrant populations. Then, I introduce nine major forms of social stress that women revealed in their life history narratives, and expound upon the meaning and interaction of these themes within the VIDDA Syndemic. While I argue that the clustering of diabetes and depression is co-constructed and understood to be interactive—even at a biological level—in this chapter I attend to the notion that the crux of their distribution is rooted in the larger political-economic and social forces from which they emerge.

Stress and Diabetes in Context

For the past thirty years medical anthropologists have developed a keen interest in cross-cultural constructions of disease, focusing specifically on the semantics of illness and suffering in various cultural milieus (Good 1977; Kleinman 1980; Nichter 1981, 2010; Kleinman 1988; Good et al. 1992; Guarnaccia 1992; Garro and Mattingly 2000; Garro 2008). For example, a seminal article by Mark Nichter (1981) describes how Havik Brahmin women use physical idioms of distress, such as menstrual pain, headaches, and back pain to communicate social disorder and emotional distress from their private lives. Peter Guarnaccia (1992) shows how Puerto Ricans use the concept of nerves, or *ataque de nervios*, to communicate anxieties and emotions associated with a social distress that is less amenable to discussion in the public sphere. Jane Poss and Mary Ann Jezewski (2002) demonstrate how Mexican Americans implicate fright, or *susto*, into explanatory models for type 2 diabetes. I have argued elsewhere that people of Mexican descent might even conceive of diabetes itself to be an idiom of distress (Mendenhall et al. 2010). In sum, these studies illustrate how individuals often link their social and emotional distress with somatic symptoms that are culturally relevant at a particular time and place.

A growing body of anthropological and public health research documents how Mexican and Mexican immigrant populations implicate susto and *coraje* (roughly translated as rage or anger) in diabetes causality (Hunt, Valenzuela, and Pugh 1998; Weller et al. 1999; Loewe and Freeman 2000; Jezewski and Poss 2002; Mercado-Martinez and Ramos-Herrera 2002; Poss and Jezewski 2002;

Neuhouser et al. 2004; Garcia et al. 2007; Mendenhall et al. 2010). For example, Mercado-Martinez and Ramos-Herrera found susto to be the most common etiologic reason for diabetes onset among low-income Mexicans in Guadalajara and describe the susto etiology as "a series of economic, social, or relational factors that produce fright in participants and together 'cause' diabetes" (2002, 797). In most cases, people link susto and diabetes etiology through acutely stressful events, such as an automobile accident, witnessing a death by gunfire or drowning, being threatened with a gun, and the sudden death of a close family member. These events often occur in the public sphere and involve family, friends, coworkers, and even strangers. In contrast, Mercado-Martinez and Ramos-Herrera found coraje, the second most common causal reasoning for diabetes onset, to arise from "social and emotional processes [that] are interconnected in such a way that when they are combined with anger and rage, they give rise to diabetes" (2002, 798). Multiple studies have documented that women report coraje more frequently than men and associate it with the private sphere, family conflict, and prolonged stressors such as domestic abuse and betrayal (Finkler 1997; Mercado-Martinez and Ramos-Herrera 2002).

Although implicating susto and coraje in diabetes causality may be rooted in Mexican culture, linking social distress to diabetes is found cross-culturally. In a multiethnic evaluation of people's beliefs about contributors to diabetes, Nancy Schoenberg and colleagues found that "without any predetermined prompting about stress and irrespective of cultural group, most informants highlighted how inadequate resources, stressful life events, and deleterious environments played a role in their diabetes" (2005, 186). Furthermore, they argued that in fact these cross-group findings proved that the stress-diabetes interface could not be relegated to a folk illness or culture-bound syndrome, such as susto. Such findings are important because when focus is placed on the unique Mexican idioms of distress, as opposed to social distress, the larger political-economic frameworks (like structural violence) that shape stressful experiences can be overlooked (Mendenhall et al. 2012).

This problem highlights a common critique in critical medical anthropology that Paul Farmer has called "immodest claims of causality" (1999, 4). This critique suggests that when social scientists emphasize cultural and psychological explanations, such as the unique aspects of folk illnesses in diabetes causality, they often overlook some of the deeply troubling contextual and structural problems that contribute to disease. This becomes problematic when such research communicates to biomedical physicians that the stress-diabetes interface might have a unique emotional component that is situated in the socio-spiritual world. As a result, these emotional idioms are classified as a form of folk belief and therefore distinct from biomedical "fact" (Good 1994).

Thus, in this chapter I focus on the social factors that women described in their life history narratives as spurring emotions such as susto, coraje, *nervios* (nerves), and *tristeza* (sadness). In doing so, I do not mean to undermine the uniquely cultural aspects of the emotional idioms central to anthropological scholarship on diabetes beliefs. Rather, I wish to emphasize the social stressors that are often contributors to and consequences of social distress, depression, and diabetes.

Narrative Themes

Based on my literature review and exploratory ethnographic research, I predicted that four overarching themes would be central to the women's stories: (1) diabetes stress, (2) gender-based violence, (3) family stress, and (4) immigration stress. Through a closer evaluation of the narrative data I better defined and broke down these codes into nine key variables that represent the most stressful and sometimes traumatic factors described in the narratives collected for this book. In the following pages I illustrate in detail common stressful experiences and deconstruct intra- and inter-thematic variations, using Domenga's and Rosie's stories as a stepping-off point.

Analysis of the narrative data revealed nine major social stressors.[1] Figure 3.1 presents these major themes according to their frequency: interpersonal abuse (65 percent), health stress (55 percent), family stress (48 percent), loss of a family member (36 percent), financial stress (35 percent), neighborhood violence (17 percent), feelings of social isolation (15 percent), immigration stress (15 percent), and work stress (15 percent). Even though I am separating these themes

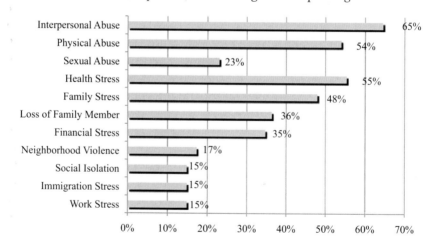

Figure 3.1   Frequency of narrative themes reported in life history narratives

for analytical purposes, a great deal of interaction exists between them. Indeed, Domenga's and Rosie's narratives exemplify how interconnections among these stressors might persist throughout the life course.

Like Domenga and Rosie, many women reported more than one narrative theme. Figure 3.2 shows the distribution of the cumulative number of stressors reported by the women in this study: all but three women reported one of the nine catalogued stresses, and the majority reported two to four different types of social stress in their life history narratives (68 percent; n = 82). While one woman reported seven of nine possible stressful experiences, the average number of stressors reported was three. In rare cases, one emotional experience was counted twice due to overlapping or concurrence of stresses (for example, if the loss of a child was associated with neighborhood violence, then both categories were recorded). In these cases, recording both categories was important due to the environmental and emotional effects that both factors had in these women's lives.

Table 3.1 displays significant correlations between social stressors. These data reveal a significant relationship between feeling socially detached and experiencing abuse, a correlation sustained with sexual abuse but not with physical abuse. There was a significant association between family discord and diabetes distress, and diabetes distress and health stress. Health stress correlated with physical abuse, but no other forms of abuse. Unsurprisingly, neighborhood stress correlated with family stress and work stress, and work stress correlated with financial stress.

These correlations will be explored in depth throughout this chapter. The remaining sections explore inter- and intra-thematic variations among the nine principal themes and discuss the role of each variable in the VIDDA Syndemic.

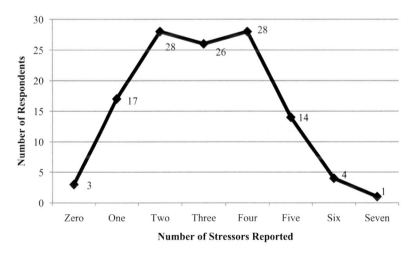

Figure 3.2 Distribution of cumulative stresses (narrative themes) reported

Table 3.1 Correlations between social stressors

Stressors	Social Isolation	Health Stress	Family Stress	Loss of Family	Neighborhood Stress	Immigration Stress	Work Stress	Financial Stress	Diabetes Distress
Abuse	0.21*	0.13	0.09	-0.12	0.07	0.07	-0.13	0	-0.1
Physical Abuse	0.16	0.20*	0.12	-0.02	0.08	0.06	-0.08	0.05	0
Sexual Abuse	0.21*	0.14	0.02	-0.09	0.01	-0.01	-0.12	-0.11	0.15
Social Isolation	-	0.1	0.25*	-0.17	-0.13	0.15	-0.04	0.13	0.20*
Health Stress	-	-	0.1	0.09	-0.03	0	0.05	-0.04	0.21*
Family Stress	-	-	-	0.17	0.26*	0.11	-0.12	0.1	0.08
Loss of Family	-	-	-	-	0.15	0.02	-0.17	-0.12	-0.03
Neighborhood Stress	-	-	-	-	-	-0.01	-0.19*	-0.15	-0.08
Immigration Stress	-	-	-	-	-	-	-0.04	-0.01	-0.09
Work Stress	-	-	-	-	-	-	-	0.23*	0.07
Diabetes Distress	-	-	-	-	-	-	-	0.14	-

Interpersonal Abuse

Two-thirds of the women who participated in this study revealed at least one form of verbal, emotional, physical, or sexual abuse. Fifty-four percent reported physical abuse, most often from a spouse or parent, and 23 percent reported sexual abuse, most often during childhood and perpetrated by a relative. The following narrative excerpts exemplify the women's descriptions of interpersonal abuse, and give a sense of how I coded verbal, emotional, physical, and sexual abuses:

[My first marriage] lasted like six and a half years and I finally left. It was—it was—it was [pause] I got beat up, almost every day. (English-speaking Mexican American woman, categorized as spousal physical abuse)

[I left my husband] because he was bad. He hit me, drank too much, didn't work, nothing. I had to care for my children. (Spanish-speaking Mexican woman, categorized as spousal physical abuse and neglect)

She [my mother] would beat us all the time for stupid things. (English-speaking Mexican American woman, categorized as childhood physical abuse)

My brothers never hit me, but my father, yes, he hit us. (Spanish-speaking Mexican women, categorized as childhood physical abuse)

He [my husband] didn't abuse me, but he scolded me a lot, especially when he drank too much. He ragged on me a lot. But sometimes, like when he was at ease, he would forget things and he wouldn't scold me. But even at these times he would rag on me a little. (Spanish-speaking Mexican woman, categorized as spousal verbal abuse)

My father, he sexually abused us. (English-speaking Mexican American woman, categorized as childhood sexual abuse)

The only thing I knew is that when my father was alive, my father used to drink a lot. [pause] And [the] only thing I remember of him is that he used to hit me. [pause] And then I knew he was, he used to carry guns and stuff and I was worried about my mom when I was young. (English-speaking Mexican American woman, categorized as childhood physical abuse)

My dad's cousin [sexually] abused me when I was small. I told my mom, but my mom didn't want to tell my dad [. . .] I was eight. (English-speaking Mexican American woman, categorized as childhood sexual abuse)

I separated from him [my first husband] because he drank too much. He would begin to drink and it made him very aggressive. On one occasion I had to call the police. He put a knife to my neck. (Spanish-speaking Mexican woman, categorized as spousal physical abuse)

My husband was very bad. I was abused. One day he was going to kill me with a knife, and he would have killed me. His brother, the husband of his sister, was the one who grabbed him and held him back. I was going to throw a chair at him, and they restrained him and let everything pass over. But he would have killed me. (Spanish-speaking Mexican woman, categorized as spousal physical abuse)

I never heard [my stepfather] swear and cuss in Spanish, but you know, he'd say that we were lazy and dirty. I can remember to this day that he would be looking out the window to make sure that my mom took the bus. Once he was sure that my mom was away, then he would go [and beat us]. He hated my brother with a passion. (English-speaking Mexican American woman, categorized as childhood physical abuse)

Physically, she [my mother] wouldn't abuse me, but mentally, she really—she really tormented me. [pause] So it was kind of rough. And if it wasn't for my sister, I don't know, you know, how I could have survived. 'Cause you know how when you cry in the nighttime for your mom, and usually your mother comes and say it's okay, you know, go back to sleep or whatever? She would wait 'til you fall asleep or give you a hug or a kiss. She never did. If she did come, she would tell me to shut up. (English-speaking Mexican American woman, categorized as childhood emotional and verbal abuse)

Linking these narrative excerpts with the current health conditions of the women who shared them provides some anecdotes for the growing body of research that suggests that interpersonal abuse, and childhood sexual and physical abuse in particular, increases one's risk for poor mental and physical health in adulthood (see Felitti et al. 1998; Shea et al. 2004). As illustrated in Domenga's and Rosie's stories, some women focused a great deal on a specific incident that had a major impact on their lives, such as childhood sexual abuse. However, stories about these experiences often ran into narratives of other types of suffering linked with other forms of abuse. For example, in the sample at large, twenty-four of the twenty-eight women (86 percent) who reported sexual abuse also reported physical abuse. And all but 10 percent of women who described verbal and/or emotional abuse also reported experiences of physical abuse, as described by the following respondent:

We suffered a great deal of poverty and I know that my mother didn't want me. And I preferred to leave the house because a man, who wasn't my boyfriend, said nothing more then, "Let's go." And I went with him and we had many children. And later he left me. [pause] And he left me with eight children and I had to work to raise them. Later I met another man and we had one child together but he gave me a bad life. He hit me a lot, a lot, a lot. All my life I have suffered. And since then he has died and I have stayed alone here with my children. (Spanish-speaking Mexican woman)

Hence, the broad interpersonal abuse category captures distinct and often overlapping forms of verbal, emotional, physical, and sexual abuse throughout the life course.

Some women articulated that they were both victims and perpetrators of interpersonal abuse. These women always described physically harming their family members as a result of anger. The following interlocutor describes her role as a perpetrator of child abuse, which she links directly with her own victimization:

The anger that I felt made me violent. Now, no, as I have learned to control it. But during that time I was very bad and it controlled me. [pause] I had these problems of being violent for fifteen years. I was unable to do anything for my children because I was like this then; it would claim me and I would use strong words. I could not stand that I was mistreated. I could not endure it, and then it would cause me to hit. I think that all of this also had something to do with the development of my diabetes and then also with the fact that my whole family has it. (Spanish-speaking Mexican woman)

The category of interpersonal abuse is an important one not only because it was so frequently reported, but also because of its connections with structural violence, symbolic violence, immigration stress, and the breakdown of social networks. The integration of these factors with interpersonal abuse was most evident in Domenga's story. Although it is the experience of sexual abuse that Domenga focuses on, we cannot overlook how the dissolution of social protections as a result of immigration, family separation, and the fear associated with undocumented status, all shaped the conditions of her father's abuse. More extreme examples of violence were Rosie's kidnapping and rape at a young age and the experience of another woman who was gang-raped at the age of ten outside her village in Mexico and left to die. She stated that her survival resulted from the mercy of one of her perpetrators, who "picked up her bloody body and brought her to town," leaving her on a neighbor's doorstep. These "invisible" capillaries of power that facilitate such violence must be recognized as accomplices to lifelong suffering and disease. Such chronic suffering cannot be dismissed, as repeated acts of subjugation—through verbal abuse, emotional manipulation, or physical battering—can become buried in the mind and manifest themselves within the body.

Health Stress

When I began open coding, I projected that diabetes stress would be a major narrative theme. Early on, however, I realized that the salience of health problems extended well beyond diabetes. Therefore, while the category of health stress incorporates diabetes talk, it is not limited to it: it also includes the stress of managing numerous physical ailments, such as chronic pain, repercussions of stroke, breast cancer, liver cancer, fibromyalgia, heart disease, and behavioral-moderated health, such as alcoholism. I adapted my goal of capturing concerns about diabetes stress to a broader goal that encompassed women's health concerns more generally.[2] I found that more than half of the women indicated their health as a major life stress (55 percent; n = 67).

Many studies of chronic disease place the highest priority—or the strongest focus—on the role of the disease in people's lives. For example, many narratives of people living with chronic disease are identified as "illness narratives," thereby giving priority to disease as a contributor to social or emotional transformation (see Kleinman 1988; Becker 1997). This study suggests that even though diabetes diagnosis might have been transformational, with time many women came to perceive diabetes to be only one of many stresses in their lives. Just as Domenga fell into a deep depression when she initially discovered her diabetes, and after many years managing the disease became accustomed to it, many women revealed that at the time we met the stress of diabetes was not central to their life stories. In other words, diabetes had become part of their everyday routine. As one woman said, "Diabetes is my friend and we must take care of one another." Some dismissed it as a problem altogether after adapting their eating and exercise routines, and others simply ignored it. Such dismissal of the struggles associated with diabetes was largely due to the fact that diabetes was but one of multiple physical health problems that women were managing and seeking treatment for at the safety-net clinic. In fact, some women suffered from social, psychiatric, and physical problems that were much more severe and potentially debilitating when compared to diabetes, such as extreme poverty, bipolar disorder, and the aftermath of stroke. Even so, many women associated the stresses of everyday life with diabetes ("Every time that I am stressed my sugars don't come down").

Diabetes, however, was the most stressful aspect of the lives of some women. This was particularly true for those women experiencing a diabetes complication,

DM
complications

such as dialysis, loss of eyesight, or amputation. Other women were fearful that some day they would develop a diabetes-related complication, and this fear was often associated with a family member's or a friend's experiences:

> I've seen people that had their legs amputated and, and stuff like that. So when I was thinking back, just thinking about how they reacted. [pause] And I'm like, oh my God, I'm going to get my legs cut off, my fingers, or whatever. You know, like my brother, he lost a toe already, so that's a starter for him. So [pause] yeah, like I said, the first year was really rough. But now it's okay. 'Cause like my [brother]—I don't think my sugar is that high. 'Cause I never seen it go up to two hundred. (English-speaking Mexican American woman)

The narratives I collected also reveal how women situated diabetes into their general medical routine, as many women were managing multiple chronic diseases at one time:

multiple chronic diseases

> [My stress is] from all of the diseases that have developed. Because imagine: I have rheumatism, diabetes, high blood pressure, and asthma. (Spanish-speaking Mexican woman)

> I started gaining lots of weight and I ended up having hypothyroid. And I think that led up to diabetes and diabetes led up to heart problems and that led up to, you know, the neuropathy and fibromyalgia and [pause] all that. (English-speaking Mexican American woman)

Some women reported that they were diagnosed with fibromyalgia. Fibromyalgia is a complicated diagnosis that characterizes those who suffer from unexplained physical symptoms (Madden and Sim 2006). The biomedical community still debates this diagnosis, as the cluster of symptoms has no clear origin and the manifestation of such pain is not uniform. However, the diagnosis itself is significant, as it can function to legitimate a person's pain, both to the self and to the social world. Because it has been argued that fibromyalgia is itself a collection of physical symptoms resulting from emotional distress (Madden and Sim 2006), it is significant that the diagnosis was mentioned by even a handful of women. I interpret this finding to be a byproduct of the high rates of psychological suffering among the women in this study and of the medical doctors' attempts to make sense of unexplained pain. The following quote exemplifies the women's narratives about fibromyalgia:

> I think those things [my fibromyalgia] come from nowhere. [pause] I don't know if it was the accident that I have on my feet and then later, like, a year later I fell again with water on a floor and they have to do surgery on both of my knees. So,

they said the fibromyalgia is triggered by, by some kind of accident, so I don't know. [pause] I just know that I suffer. (English-speaking Mexican American woman)

Besides mentioning that they were diagnosed with the disorder, or describing briefly their symptoms, women did not go into detail about their experiences coping with fibromyalgia. Even so, the significance of fibromyalgia—a diagnosis of chronic physical pain, or somatic disorder—provides an important area for future study that may unfold the interconnection between such severe psychological and social suffering and chronic disease. Because physical pain is associated with emotions and psychosocial factors in complex ways, it may be that fibromyalgia functions as a *medical* idiom for far more extreme psychological suffering and as a way to provide medical services for women who report severely traumatic histories.

I incorporated substance abuse into this category of health stress because all of the women who reported substance abuse also reported a current physical problem. In most cases, women described substance abuse—from heroin to alcohol, cigarettes, and marijuana—as a problem of the past. In the present, these substances were often described as part of their social world, meaning that even if they were not using them, these substances affected them as a result of a loved one's abuse. Most women did not currently drink, smoke, or use drugs; if they did in the past, they attributed their cessation of such activities to older age, and some specifically attributed it to diabetes. A limited number of women reported ongoing struggles with substance abuse, as illustrated by the following forty-year-old U.S.-born woman suffering from severe bipolar disorder, severe diabetes, and alcoholism:

> A lot of times I black out and then I get in arguments with my husband. [pause] But then he would be drinking at the same time too. [pause] So, it's, I mean we'd just get started, and just [pause] days just become a blur. (English-speaking Mexican American woman)

Finally, this narrative theme does not necessarily capture psychiatric distress. To isolate the impact of psychiatric distress, which transversed all the narrative themes and was a frequent component of women's life stories, I employed validated inventories of depression, post-traumatic stress disorder, and diabetes distress. However, I must emphasize that while "health stress" measured the women's mentions of *physical* pain, such aspects of well-being were rarely dissociated from emotional pain or social stress. Moreover, within this population of low-income Mexican immigrant women, prolonged physical health problems were the corollary of structural problems. This was because the delay in seeking health care played a role in the severity of women's health complications, and such delay may be attributed to poverty or lack of documentation. It was also

[margin annotation: substance use / abuse]

a result of limited access to affordable medications, weakened social networks, and untenable institutional support (such as language barriers), which may have increased the stress of chronic disease management for many. In this sense, social and structural problems and emotional and social well-being were fundamental in how women experienced "health".

Family Stress

The family was a tightly woven thread throughout many women's life stories. They recounted events from their pasts through a recollection of family relation-ships and communicated a sense of identity rooted in the family itself. Almost half of the women I met (n = 58) described the high-risk behaviors, chronic ill-nesses, and persistent needs of their family members as central to their current life stress. Many of these women placed the needs of family members before their own. The principal role of other people's worries in women's life stories is important not only because it might hinder the women's ability to acknowledge and accept negative emotions associated with personal suffering, but also because prioritizing the stress of others can be a barrier to diabetes self-care.

Women primarily reported family stress in relation to their role as caretakers of elderly parents, sick siblings, mischievous children, and grandchildren, and/or as wives of unfaithful, sick, or drug-abusing husbands:

I tried to explain to my brother, I need help. I need help with her [my sister]. She gets mad. It's not normal the way she gets mad, and, like I said, he's in his own little world. And he didn't believe me—he thought I was exaggerating. My sister also thought I was exaggerating, but they weren't living with her. So then I finally told him, I said you gotta come over here and see her, and then he realized, yeah, and then he was in our life for all the time she was sick. And, since she passed, he went back to the way he was before. (English-speaking Mexican American woman)

I have like, financial stress, and stress at home. [pause] 'Cause watching my mom and my grandma—taking care of—being with two older women, it just—really, it's very stressful. Like, taking care of them, their medical problems. Their everyday daily activi-ties, especially with my mother 'cause she's obese too. And just getting her like, well let's go do this, and then it's like my grandma comes in and she's very negative and she's just like, no, no. [pause] And so we just wind up not doing nothing. It's just like things like that, that just kind of adds to it. (English-speaking Mexican American)

In addition, women worried a great deal about their children, and this stress played a major role in their lives. This aspect of their narratives was not unexpected, as 90 percent of my interlocutors were mothers. Thirty percent had five or more children, and often women lived with and depended upon their children financially. A small percentage of them had children, parents, or siblings living with and depending on them financially. In some cases, women were currently providing care for their adolescent or adult children—for example, if a child was a minor or had mental or physical disabilities. In other cases, my interlocutors worried about their children's struggles and involvement with gangs or drugs on the streets of Chicago.

> I am sad because of my life, because of my kids. Because I have one daughter who has problems: she lost her house, she has a child with Down's Syndrome, she lost her car, she has to move from Texas to here because she lost her job, she was in debt. They lost everything. (Spanish-speaking Mexican woman)

> I don't know what happened to my daughter. She's just totally opposite of the boys. She's literally hazardous to my health, she cannot live in my household. A few years ago, she begged me to move in, in an apartment in Carol Stream with her and I'm like, we can't live together. "No ma, I'm not gonna drink, I'm not gonna get high— you know—I'm gonna be good." I'm like [pause] I gave in. I went to [the town] with her. She started drinking and getting high again. She had my blood pressure so high, the doctor doubled my dosage, gave me an extra pill. He goes, if you don't calm down you're gonna have stroke or a nervous breakdown. And it got to the point where I'm like, you're [pause] I'm not gonna end up in jail. [pause] 'Cause I just wanted to choke her. And I'm like, Tanya [pseudonym], don't push my buttons. I go, "You underestimate me. You know, back up." And she got in my face. "Mom, I don't wanna box with you." And I busted out laughing. I go, "Tanya, there's not gonna be no boxing involved. If I get my hands on you girl, it's gonna be all over." I go, "There's nobody here to stop me." I go, "The only reason I haven't grabbed you is because I just might kill you before somebody gets here." I go, "That's the only reason I haven't grabbed you." (English-speaking Mexican American woman)

Finally, women spoke of their troubles with their husbands. Thirty-nine percent of the women were currently married (n = 47), often to second or third husbands, 7 percent lived with a domestic partner (n = 9), 35 percent were divorced (n = 42), 8 percent were widowed (n = 10), and 11 percent never married (n = 13). The category of family stress does not capture interpersonal abuse (seen above), but rather the strain associated to a family member's behavior. Specifically, a male partner's involvement in gang- or drug-related activities was a major stressor for many women:

> He [my husband] was just an abuser to himself. Um, no abuse to his children, no abuse to me. It's just that he cared more about that drug than he did about the family having food on the table or money for necessities. So I started working. I said, dear God get me off of this and I will go to work everyday whether I'm sick or not.

And I got my first job. [pause] I didn't know what I was getting myself into. He [my husband] is known as an addict. Drug addict. He has been on the methadone clinic, which I don't understand why it's been so long, ever since my son was born, and my son is thirty-eight years old. That's how long he's been on the methadone clinic. And now that he's like sixty-five, he says he wants to quit and quit and quit. I just think that I just grew up and I didn't like it, I grew tired. One year I said, I'm gonna go on my own. He didn't know, nobody knew, not even my kids, where I moved to, just my mom and my sister. And one year, nobody knew where I lived my life. And I liked it. (English-speaking Mexican American woman)

Embedding the self within the larger context of the family has significance for women, and particularly for people with diabetes. Cultural models of gendered behavior place women at the center of the home, as nurturer, caregiver, and food-preparer, which have traditionally been considered "women's work" in patriarchal societies on both sides of the Mexican–U.S. border (Finkler 1994, 1997; Hirsch 2003a; Farr 2006; Sciolla et al. 2011). While these social roles may indeed be changing as a consequence of immigration (Hirsch 2003a), it is clear that many women feel that their role as family caregivers is central to their identity and everyday life. At the same time, there is a tension between social expectations for women to care for the family and their diabetes, which requires them to change the diet, increase physical activity, monitor blood glucose, and take medicines regularly (Fisher et al. 2000). Many women explained that because they commonly prepared food for and ate with family members without diabetes, modifying their diets would require their immediate family to do so. This statement put the culpability of their own diabetes self-care in the hands of family members, and therefore reduced or excused blame for poor diabetes management.

Subsequent chapters will reveal that family stress alone was not significantly associated with depression or PTSD. Yet, this narrative theme intersects with stresses associated with domestic violence, poverty, chronic illness, immigration, and neighborhood violence, and, perhaps most importantly, it strongly correlated with reporting feelings of social isolation (see Table 3.1 above). Family stress breaches these categories as a direct reflection of the women's beliefs that caretaking is a primary role for them within the family; interestingly, perhaps the strongest determinant of distress was when women felt detached from the family that they prioritized so highly.

Feeling Social Isolated

A small subset of women described deep-seated feelings of social isolation and loneliness in their daily lives. Eighteen women (15 percent) mentioned these feelings, of which sixteen were born in Mexico and two in the United States. Many of the Mexican-born women reported longing for their families in Mexico while at the same time feeling lonely and misunderstood by their children with whom they resided in the United States. The importance of understanding the impact of these troubling feelings on health is underscored in research demonstrating the links between social isolation and health (Berkman and Syme 1979; Berkman et al. 2000). Further, this category proved to be one of the most powerful predictors of depression (see chapter 5).

Social detachment was often described in generational terms. Many of the late-adult women in this study found solace in a sister, a friend, or someone else who was within their age range. Many of the women who reported feelings of social isolation spoke to a deep longing for someone who understood them, someone who was their social contemporary. The following narrative excerpt exemplifies this thematic category:

> My sisters are in Mexico and when I speak to them we talk about other things, many things. Yes, I lived there many years ago. Since my mother died I didn't return for a long time. My mother died in '78 and I didn't return to see them [my sisters] until '96. This is what has made my life very difficult. (Spanish-speaking Mexican woman)

Interestingly, in rare cases women relayed that they felt taken advantage of since moving to United States, as they believed their grown children expected them to care for the house, cooking, and childcare. Some said that they felt trapped now that they were in Chicago and often longed for friends and family in Mexico:

> [I came here when I was] forty-five. I came here to be here with my two daughters. Nothing else. I should have stayed there [in Mexico]. I wouldn't have developed diabetes. But the good Lord says this. And you can repeat what I say, Señorita. What is done is done. My nieces all wanted me to come. I told them, what if I come and I die? [She is very frightened of the weather and blames it as the cause of her diabetes.] They say to me, "You will be with us, Auntie, you will be with us. Come and see, Auntie, we want you to come here with us." And sometimes I feel like leaving [and returning to Mexico]. And my kids say to me, "No, where would you go?" They say that because who is going to cook, who is going to look after the [kids]? [pause] No, no. Yes, I want to go. I am already tired of the cold, I can't leave the house in all this snow. (Spanish-speaking Mexican woman)

While some women came out and simply stated, "I'm lonely," most women described this sentiment by sharing a longing for another time or place. This narrative theme was clearly a byproduct of the migratory experience: women spoke of longing not for Mexican food or culture, but rather for the companionship of close friends and family who understood them and their needs. At the same time, they felt that their family in the United States, often children and grandchildren, didn't understand them. Acknowledging these feelings of loneliness and isolation from their family and friends in Chicago might have been especially important for the women who reported this narrative theme because many of these women concurrently reported sexual abuse (see Table 3.1), and their isolating themselves might be associated with harboring a difficult memory or secret from their children. I will unpack this narrative theme further in the following chapter as I discuss how feeling a part of the social fabric on both sides of the Mexico–U.S. border is fundamental to mental health. Through its intimate connection to immigration experiences, therefore, feeling socially detached plays a unique role in the VIDDA Syndemic.

Loss of a Family Member

When conducting life history interviews, I hypothesized that the loss of a family member would strongly correlate with depression. This belief was rooted in the emotional narratives shared by just over one in four women (27 percent; n = 33) interviewed who addressed the loss of a parent, spouse, sibling, or child. While all women had likely lost someone, only some discussed this loss in their life stories. Unsurprisingly, the most emotive narratives were associated with recent loss. Such mortality was attributed to old age, freak accidents, gun violence, suicide, poor health, and diabetes.

These stories often relayed a profound disruption in the woman's social life, in addition to major financial and emotional deficits. For example, Domenga's husband's death not only was an emotional struggle, but also influenced her economic situation. At the time of his death, Domenga was raising two young children and depended on her husband completely for financial security. After his death, Domenga had to rely on the support of her mother and sister and to reenter the public-sphere working world. Many women described similar narratives of grief associated with the loss of parents, siblings, or children with whom they were very close. Such loss had an impact on their social worlds, their everyday lives, and their family members' lives, as illustrated by the following quote:

> I was depressed after my father died in '07. For, like, seven months. I was like, very depressed. 'Cause you know, I was the one that's taking care of him, and I felt that, you know, I could have done a better job. (English-speaking Mexican American woman)

When I lost my granddaughter, I got [pause] I don't know how—what you would call it? I got very angry with God. I got different ideas of him, and I still do. In fact I had them a long time, but I tried to go along with the program and think he's great and loving, I really do try to make myself think of that, but when I think of things that go on, it's hard of me to think like that. You understand what I'm saying? Like he's good and great and loving [pause] and then all these things happen. (English-speaking Mexican American woman who lost her granddaughter to leukemia three months before the interview)

Some women struggled with the loss of a loved one to diabetes. This was particularly troubling because it made them think, and certainly worry, about their own diabetes problems.

Yeah, that was bad. [pause] Then my sister, my youngest sister, she just passed away last Sunday. She had diabetes all her life, and it took everything. She was amputated. She had a brain tumor, she went blind, took her teeth. She was a big woman, you know, and she end up being eighty pounds. [Last week] she had a heart attack, and then a massive heart attack. (English-speaking Mexican American woman)

My youngest sister's in very bad shape with her diabetes. And that's what my brother died of—my youngest brother. (English-speaking Mexican American woman)

The following respondent describes how the recent loss of her adult daughter to diabetes was a profoundly harrowing experience for her. This short excerpt gives only a glimpse of the emotional state this women was in; she cried so much throughout the interview that she was at times difficult to understand.

I believe my daughter was thirty-six. She died three months ago from diabetes. Her sugar dropped too low when she was sleeping in the basement and her boyfriend didn't notify me in time. When I went to see her she had too much phlegm in her throat from the low blood sugar. [pause] I couldn't do anything. (Spanish-speaking Mexican woman)

The recent loss of a family member frequently resulted in coping mechanisms such as crying alone and sheltering emotions from others (particularly family members). This mechanism was commonly reported when my interlocutors discussed life's most distressing events, but the women's coping strategies varied greatly. Some women were, like Domenga, able to face each struggle as it comes, to "pick up her luggages and go on in life again." Oftentimes this perspective was communicated by women who were surrounded by family and felt responsibility for and support from them. As I described in the previous section, some women described feeling isolated and alone. This sentiment influenced coping mechanisms because many of these women's confidants (specifically those of their generation, mostly sisters) lived in Mexico or elsewhere in the United States, while my respondents lived in Chicago with their children. In addition, not being able to attend the funeral of a loved one in Mexico because of lack of documentation was a common grievance for those who were unauthorized immigrants.

Even though such loss was mentioned several times throughout women's narratives, the lack of association between loss of a loved one and depression in unadjusted analyses (presented in chapter 5) revealed that such loss was not fundamental to psychiatric distress. This lack of association held true even when examining the narratives of those who experienced recent loss (which represented 12 percent of women) or loss of a child (15 percent). However, the loss of a family member, particularly when recent, obviously affected the woman's social support system, economic security, and therefore overall mental distress. This is particularly relevant in the case of the loss of the primary breadwinner, as in Domenga's case. Thus, even though the loss of a loved one was not corollary to VIDDA Syndemic interaction, it was a central component of the life stories of many women.

Financial Stress

All of the women in this study were poor, and 80 percent were living below the poverty line. One in three women (n = 42) identified financial troubles as a cause of chronic stress in their life stories. These women were more likely to have completed a higher level of education and to have held a job compared to the women who did not mention financial struggles. Interestingly, a crude bivariate logistic regression analysis indicates that women who had attended some secondary school (n = 51) were 1.90 times (p < 0.10) more likely to report financial stress when compared to women who did not finish, or attend, primary school (n = 70). This finding may be a result of the fact that women with higher levels of education were more likely to work in the public sphere, manage their personal finances, and therefore worry about the financial state of the family. In contrast, women with much less education were more likely to live with family members in a shared family complex (if they were not living with their children) and to work primarily in the domestic domain. Further, more educated women might have higher expectations for financial well-being or be more aware of their relative poverty compared to women with limited formal schooling.

This narrative theme, therefore, measures the subjective stress associated with lack of access to financial resources, and poverty more generally. The following excerpts exemplify the women's stories about financial stress as a principal cause of disorder in their lives:

> I think mostly it was the economic stress. I think 'cause it was, when you don't know how you're gonna survive, 'cause see the problem we have, my husband lost his job and he had a good job. So the company closed down. So that was very stressful. I was in real estate at that time [and] was struggling too; so I was not doing anything. He was doing nothing. So we started getting unemployment compensation. Well we're not used to it—this is the first time he applied and we been here the same time over forty years. (English-speaking Mexican American woman)

> I feel a little worried about my situation right now because I have so many bills for food, for bus fair, and my sales [in my job] are not good. (Spanish-speaking Mexican woman)

> My job is very exhausting. The job is very hard but to a certain point you have to be okay with it because it is going to help your family, give you money. At this time I made $3.35 per hour, very little. There was never much money, never enough money that I was making because I had to pay the rent and the bills—I had personal expenses, too, and I paid them. (Spanish-speaking Mexican woman)

If this study were repeated, I would inquire about food insecurity and the difficulties women faced in accessing healthy and affordable foods. This problem certainly bears weight on the women's overall health, including obesity, and specifically diabetes self-care (such as maintaining a healthy diet). However, this was a theme that emerged peripherally, so I did not include it in my analysis. The following excerpt demonstrates one woman's struggle to access and consume healthy and safe foods:

> Yeah, my fridge don't work. My friend buys me the food. She usually buys me the fruits and stuff and she'll buy me what I need to eat. Because the stove don't work and then I have to use the electric pot and it takes forever to cook because if I don't eat right away I end up shaking and I know that I have to eat. It makes me feel bad because all my food is getting all spoiled. [pause] Every time I buy it the food is already spoiled within two or three days. Then like I said sometimes, I, you know, I wonder if it's good or not good and then I end up getting sick. (English-speaking Mexican American woman)

The issue of food availability also arose when the women discussed their struggles to maintain the healthy diets advised by their doctors. Many women stated that maintaining the diabetic diet was simply impossible due to the structural constraints they faced. Underscored by the term "food deserts," availability, affordability, and access to healthy and safe food is fundamental to understanding epidemic cycles of diabetes, stress, and structural violence in poor urban environments. Food deserts are neighborhoods that are peppered with small convenience stores and fast-food establishments but have limited access to groceries that provide fresh produce. This geospatial problem of grocer distribution in Chicago is a major barrier to the knowledge and consumption of healthy foods among the poor (see Beaulac, Kristjansson, and Cummins 2009). Food deserts represent a critical form of structural violence insofar as the structure of neighborhoods and organization of cities literally shape individuals' access to healthy foods.

Work Stress

One in every six women described work-related stress, such as perceived racism in the workplace, as a significant disturbance (n = 18). The salience of work-related grievances holds particular importance because only one-quarter of the sample worked outside the home (n = 33). While one quarter (n = 30) of the women stated that they were homemakers (who never worked outside the home), another quarter reported that they were disabled (n = 31), and 16 percent (n = 20) were unemployed. The remainder were retired or students.

Among the smaller number of those who were currently or previously employed, women reported having experienced a great deal of stress either as a result of a current job or as a past stressor that had contributed to lifetime cumulative stress, because of work-related injuries, racism, or unfair compensation. Such experiences are captured by the following narrative excerpts:

> When I was working for Fannie Mae there was too much stress, too much pressure. The job was very fast, there were many problems. And there, since I was having to work there, I think that I developed hypertension, and that was because of the pace of the job. I was packing chocolates, packing one chocolate and putting it into a box. And it was very—the boxes just passed so quickly. (Spanish-speaking Mexican woman)

> In my job there are injustices. There are injustices. I have a restriction; right now they say I am disabled, permanently. I am not able to lift heavy things, I am not able to push more than ten pounds, and they abuse this. Yesterday she [my boss] was like, there was an abuse that involved me, therefore she told our supervisor that she gave me a warning, and that I wasn't heeding her. I saw her. But I said to her, I said, I am not one to keep quiet. But they all came out and they wanted to talk with her. I spoke the language perfectly. Then I said to the woman, help me, and I discussed with her. I told her many things, many points that were not right. They say they

abused me, because I had a restriction. This is not in the computer. Neither am I going to put it on a sign here. I have two dislocated discs, had two foot surgeries, and now my knees hurt and I fall a lot. I am suffering a lot. My doctor looked at me and put three injections in my back. He told me that I was permanently disabled. But the company still calls me and calls me to work. They said to me that they saw the restriction, but they don't have to respect the restriction. [pause] It is because I am Mexican and because you are Filipino-American, I said—and you don't say anything about the blacks. She apologized to me and it looked very bad. (Spanish-speaking Mexican woman)

Work stress played a more prominent role in the narratives relayed by women working outside the home in Chicago, as opposed to the larger number of women who worked within the home. Specifically, women working in the public sphere reported feeling persecuted for their race and documentation status by people outside of their social network, including managers and people apart from their coethnic group. On the one hand, undocumented women related the fear of being identified by immigration while at work and being deported (either themselves or family members). On the other hand, documented women described the stress of being displaced at work because an undocumented person was willing to receive less pay and would not require government benefits. In both cases, women felt stressed and persecuted because of racism or language-based discrimination at work. In addition, many women lamented the financial burden of losing their job, factory work in particular, as their diabetes symptoms advanced.

Neighborhood Violence

Seventeen percent of women expressed distress associated with living in a neighborhood with high rates of crime, which fostered feelings of fear and insecurity. The problem of neighborhood violence can be understood as a byproduct of structural violence, immigration, and urban segregation, which are all fundamental to the VIDDA Syndemic. Women often discussed problems of neighborhood violence in relation to their children's membership in, potential involvement in, or even interaction with local gangs.

One of my sons behaved very badly. He was in a gang. Because of this I felt very tired, very desperate, very angry, very desperate. At that time I worked from six in the morning to six in the afternoon, and by the time I reached my house I would have to go look for him in the park. I did not sleep at all. I worried a lot about him. Too much. I cried and until this time he continues in the same way. (Spanish-speaking Mexican woman)

Other women described ways in which gang- or drug-related violence had a direct impact on their family's life. The most extreme narratives involved children who died as a result of crossfire, or a son who hung himself as a result of gang-related threats.

Fear of such neighborhood violence extended to individual behavior and diabetes self-care, as well. Many women feared walking alone in neighborhood parks due to the threat of gang activity, and they cited this problem as the primary reason that they did not follow the exercise routine recommended by their primary care physicians.

> We weren't afraid of walking in the street, back in the days. Now, you can't walk in the—not even half block and you're being attacked, raped, killed, you know—here in Chicago it is [pause] I don't go out here in Chicago. (English-speaking Mexican American woman)

Interestingly, fear and grief associated with neighborhood violence were more commonly noted by English-speaking women born in the United States compared to Spanish-speaking women born in Mexico. For example, sixteen of the twenty-one women (76 percent) who reported this narrative theme were English speaking, and most lived in mixed ethnic neighborhoods such as Logan Square, Uptown, and South Chicago, as opposed to predominantly Mexican immigrant neighborhoods such as Pilsen and Little Village. While these data are not conclusive, this finding substantiates research that documents lower rates of overall street crime and higher levels of social cohesion and institutional support in Mexican enclave neighborhoods as opposed to multiethnic neighborhoods in Chicago (Sampson, Morenoff, and Gannon-Rowley 2002; Morenoff, Sampson, and Raudenbush 2006). The fact that it was more common for English-speaking women living in more ethnically diverse neighborhoods to complain of the influence of drugs and gang-related violence in their lives may reflect a greater trend of dissolution of fundamental social networks and support systems among second-generation immigrants who live apart from more insular immigrant communities. This narrative theme may therefore be intimately connected with immigration stress and the larger experience of structural violence and clustering of social, psychological, and physical problems among first- and second-generation Mexican immigrants, which are reflected in all aspects of the VIDDA Syndemic.

Immigration Stress

This final narrative theme holds important leverage in the VIDDA Syndemic. Two-thirds of the women interviewed (n = 79) were born in Mexico and immigrated to Chicago at some point, most often during adolescence or early adulthood.[3] Their immigration experiences varied, including both documented and undocumented immigration, and, in some cases, seasonal migration to the United States from Mexico. Some of the women born in Chicago also reported stress related to the immigration status of their husbands and other family members, thereby demonstrating that immigration also had an impact on their lives through people close to them. One in every six women, and almost one in four of first-generation immigrants, mentioned some form of immigration-related stress as central to their life stories (n = 18).

Although undocumented women were unsurprisingly reticent about discussing their legal status while the recorder was turned on, the final survey question of the mixed-methods interview addressed documentation status. Of the women interviewed, 60 percent (n = 72) reported that they were citizens and 40 percent (n = 49) reported that they were not. Of these women who were not citizens, 67 percent (n = 33) were undocumented. There may have been some hesitance to share this information, and the rates of undocumented status may have been slightly higher than these findings reveal. Moreover, this question failed to capture the number of women who were undocumented upon arrival to the United States who subsequently gained authorization. Based on their life stories, the number of women who immigrated without documentation was most likely much higher than the number of women who were undocumented at the time we met.

Most immigration stress stories included within this narrative theme were related to documentation status, and specifically to problems associated with deportation, as illustrated by the following narrative excerpts:

> They took my son to jail and gave him to immigration. They caught him driving, and I am not sure why, and then they gave him his rights and passed him over to immigration. So it was a great deal of anxiety to think that—they had a child, and they went to go and put him there. He didn't know what to do next. And they put him in jail [for three months] and that was it. (Spanish-speaking Mexican woman)

> One [of my two brothers] is a year older than me, he lives in Mexico. He used to live here, but he did something and they deported him. And there's another one. He's like three years older than me. [pause] He was deported, too. (English-speaking Mexican American woman)

While documentation-related stress after relocating to the United States was common, women also emphasized stressful and sometimes traumatic experiences related to immigration itself. Like Domenga, those women who immigrated by foot (rather than by bus or plane, which suggests that they had a visa) frequently revealed traumatic memories associated with their actual immigration experiences, such as crossing the border in the dark and feeling like their lives were in danger. Some women who had immigrated on their own reported that they went to extremes to arrive to the United States, and that these experiences were profoundly difficult:

> Immigration? It was very hard—almost too difficult to remember. First we passed through the river, and when they [coyotes] brought us to the river, they told us that they could kill us. We could do what we wanted, but there was nobody there to hear us. And that is how we passed through the river. And then there was a companion who was with me who now I consider my son. We went together because I was drowning: I couldn't keep my head above water and then my feet couldn't hold me up. He grabbed me [. . .]
>
> [Later that night he took us to a bar] and for me it was very hard because never in my life had I been to a bar, or taken another person there. It was there where my brother violated my daughter. It was such a terrible thing that I ran [from the bar]. I ran with my cousins, and told immigration that I had no papers. (Spanish-speaking Mexican woman)

This excerpt exemplifies how the structural and interpersonal vulnerability associated with undocumented status produces profoundly negative circumstances for women and children. In the case above, this vulnerability was perpetuated further by the inequal relationship between the *coyote* and the woman on the one hand, and the woman's brother and her daughter on the other; these interpersonal sources of violence are particularly egregious and haunting in one's memory.

The impact of immigration stress on women's lives extends well beyond the ways in which this narrative theme was measured. Domenga's life story illustrates how prominently immigration-related stress can shape one's experiences: as a childhood stress related to growing up in a transnational family, as a lack of social support and legal protection related to her father's abuse, and as a legacy of financial strain related to her husband's premature death (and lack of documentation). Moreover, while not always so explicit, the actual migratory experience itself was an underlying contributor to stress in many women's lives.

To understand how immigration experiences might intersect with other social stresses, I correlated them with four discrete markers of immigration (see Table 3.2). These data must be interpreted closely, based on the directionality of the immigration marker. Positive correlations with language, birthplace, and undocumented status must be understood to indicate a higher incidence of a given stressor among women who are Spanish-speaking, born in Mexico, and

Table 3.2 Correlations of stresses with immigration measures

Stressor	Birthplace	Language Preference	Acculturation	Undocumented Status
Interpersonal Abuse	−0.21*	−0.16	0.22**	−0.13
Physical Abuse	−0.29***	−0.19*	0.30***	−0.21*
Sexual Abuse	−0.18*	−0.18*	0.23**	−0.16
Social Isolation	0.21*	0.26**	−0.28**	0.11
Health Stress	0.01	0.04	−0.09	−0.01
Family Stress	0.01	−0.07	0.03	−0.03
Loss of Family	−0.1	−0.07	0.12	−0.12
Neighborhood Stress	−0.12	−0.26	0.24**	−0.08
Immigration Stress	0.26**	0.26**	−0.33***	0.21*
Work Stress	−0.04	−0.11	0.09	−0.15
Financial Stress	0.06	0.07	−0.02	−0.06
Diabetes Distress	0.02	0.03	−0.03	0.04

*$p \leq 0.05$; **$p \leq 0.01$; ***$p \leq 0.001$.

undocumented, respectively. In contrast, positive correlations with acculturation (such as the adhesion to the dominant values of the new environment—see next chapter) indicate a higher incidence of a particular stressor among those who hold U.S. values and beliefs, as opposed to Mexican values and beliefs.[4] For example, the positive correlation between social isolation and birthplace indicates that first-generation Mexican immigrant women were more likely to report such feelings. The opposite is true for revealing a history of interpersonal abuse. In fact, reporting interpersonal abuse correlated strongly with being second-generation Mexican American (both English speaker and born in the United States). There is also a strong positive correlation between acculturation and neighborhood violence, underscoring the potential link between neighborhood cohesion and immigrant enclaves. In addition, there was a significant association between being undocumented immigrants and immigration stress. These findings and the role of immigration stress in women's life stories, independently and together with depression and diabetes, will be discussed in more depth in the next chapter.

Unpacking VIDDA

Unpacking VIDDA requires that we evaluate the social realities of women's lives. Indeed, attending to the emotional dimensions of people's lives, both at the social and individual level, is what makes this a study of syndemics instead of a microcosmic analysis of the diabetes epidemic. I conclude with three key points that stem from the data presented so far.

First, the high prevalence of interpersonal abuse suggests that the conditions in which women live may increase the risk for and experience of abuse. Specifically, reports of interpersonal abuse were substantially more frequent among my interlocutors when compared to those cited in studies of Mexican Americans diverse in socioeconomic status. For example, Lown and Vega (2001) found a 10.7 percent prevalence of physical abuse in a socioeconomically diverse population of Mexican American women, compared to the 54 percent of my interlocutors. My findings, indeed, resemble those of a study focused on a similarly impoverished group of Mexican immigrant women seeking primary care at a safety-net clinic in California: more than half of the women in that study reported physical violence (Heilemann, Kury, and Lee 2005). It is crucial to identify such intraethnic differences because they demonstrate that high rates of interpersonal abuse may stem from contextual factors, such as poverty and immigration stress (see Benson et al. 2004), as opposed to Mexican or Mexican American ethnicity. While there certainly are cultural factors that contribute to the manner in which individuals cope with and manage stress, the distribution of such social distress at the population level must be understood as a consequence of structural inequalities. As such, interpersonal abuse, which is often gender-based, may be understood to be one manifestation of such inequities (Bourgois 2009).

Second, on average the women in this study reported two to four major life stressors, and many of the narrative themes were correlated with one another. Understanding the interactions and effects of two or more stresses in the life course is essential, as we have learned that stressful experiences rarely occur in isolation (Dong et al. 2004). For example, while the broad category of interpersonal abuse correlated strongly with feelings of social isolation, there was some variability between physical and sexual abuse. Sexual abuse strongly correlated with those feelings, but physical abuse did not. Such findings might suggest that women who have experienced sexual abuse are more likely to isolate from arterial social networks. Also, because sixteen of the eighteen women who reported feelings of social isolation were Mexican immigrants, it may be that changing familial, cultural, and social structures affect coping strategies linked with interpersonal abuse. At the same time, many of these women reported more general family stress, which may figure into their tendency to isolate socially, in addition to their diabetes distress. Such findings may further indicate that these women are less likely to seek support from family and friends for their emotional needs or diabetes care.

Third, through an examination of these narrative themes, the macrolevel political, economic, and social inequalities that facilitate these microlevel stresses become clearer. For example, financial stress and the breakdown of social networks resulting from immigration played a powerful role in cultivating the conditions in which women experienced abuse and social detachment. At the same time, women described everyday struggles with economic insecurity, work stress, and family stress. They communicated fears rooted in the deleterious environments in which they lived, often linking gang- and drug-related violence with family stress and immigration stress. In addition, many immigrant women feared every day for the safety of their family members, while at the same time they struggled with family discord. Understanding these interconnections is fundamental to the VIDDA Syndemic because it is the confluence of structural violence, poverty, and stress together that contributes to the significant burden of depression and diabetes within this population.

In conclusion, the microlevel stresses exposed in this chapter demonstrate the ways in which chronic, everyday stress might manifest itself in depression and diabetes. The everyday struggles revealed by the women in this study must be understood to be interlinked with the increasing diabetes problem among socially disadvantaged groups in the United States because these stresses shape the ways in which people interact with their environment. Moreover, the women's narratives reveal how these nine factors increase the risk of diabetes through poor eating habits, physical inactivity, depression, and importantly, obesity. Thus, understanding the social complexities behind the VIDDA Syndemic is critical for realizing how everyday experiences shape mental distress and bodily suffering.

4

BORDERLANDS:
IMMIGRATION, INTEGRATION, AND ISOLATION

In *Borderlands* Gloria Anzaldúa writes:

> Faceless, nameless, invisible, taunted with "hey cucaracho" (cockroach). Trembling with fear, yet filled with courage, a courage born of desperation. Barefoot and uneducated, Mexicans with hands like boot soles gather at night by the river where two worlds merge creating what Reagan calls a frontline, a war zone [. . .] The Mexican woman is especially at risk. Often the coyote (smuggler) doesn't feed her for days or let her go to the bathroom. He often rapes her or sells her into prostitution. She cannot call on county or state health or economic resources because she doesn't know English and she fears deportation. American employers are quick to take advantage of her helplessness. She can't go home. She's sold her house, her furniture, borrowed from friends in order to pay the coyote who charges her four or five thousand dollars to smuggle her to Chicago. She may work as a live-in maid for white, Chicano, or Latino Households for as little as $15 a week. Or work in the garment industry, do hotel work. Afraid of getting caught and deported, living with as many as fifteen people in one room, the Mexicana suffers serious health problems. (1987, 33–34)

Gloria Anzaldúa introduces the plight of many Mexican immigrant women who experience challenges incomprehensible to mainstream America, both during the migration from their homes in Mexico to Chicago and during the subsequent days, months, and years living as immigrants in Chicago. Despite

81

"Latino
Health
Paradox"

such extreme psychological and social suffering, Mexicans who immigrate to Chicago are all-around healthier when compared to those born in Chicago and the United States at large. This phenomenon is widely known as the "Latino Health Paradox," as it is considered contradictory that despite coming from a poorer nation, immigrants maintain lower all-cause mortality rates when compared to their U.S.-born counterparts (Lara et al. 2005). Interestingly, the longer immigrants live in the United States, the worse their health becomes. These trends hold up for both diabetes (Borrell et al. 2009; Cowie et al. 2010; Pabon-Nau et al. 2010) and depression (Gonzalez et al. 2009).

Many scholars argue that the worsening of health among immigrants and their children is the fault of culture. As immigrants adopt the cultural habits, traits, and ideals of a new population (a phenomenon known as "acculturation"), they lose some, if not all, of the traits they previously held. A large body of social science research has explored the relationship between acculturation and health outcomes. These studies suggest that cultural adjustments play a role in changes in diet and activity patterns (Arcia et al. 2001; Abraido-Lanza, Chao, and Flórez 2005), stress and emotional coping styles (Farley et al. 2005), and cohesion with the coethnic group (Eschbach et al. 2004). As such, this scholarship suggests that these cultural changes have a major impact on key "risk factors" of poor health, such as poor diet (Marks, Garcia, and Solis 1990; Guendelman and Abrams 1995; Bermudez, Falcon, and Tucker 2000; Dixon, Sundquist, and Winkleby 2000; Neuhouser et al. 2004), obesity (Popkin and Udry 1998; Gordon-Larsen et al. 2003), and mental distress (Moscicki et al. 1989; Escobar, Hoyos Nervi, and Gara 2000; Hovey and Magana 2000). However, few studies have explored in depth the roles of immigration, social isolation, and individual struggles for social integration as major factors contributing to the Latino health paradox.

The main goal of this chapter is to examine the social factors associated with the immigration experiences that contribute to mental and physical health. First, I juxtapose the debate surrounding the Latino Health Paradox in social psychology and medical anthropology. Second, I introduce Mari's narrative to explore how social distress can result from immigration itself. I follow anthropologists Sarah Willen, Heide Castañeda, and others to discuss Mari's narrative through an examination of the dynamic, synergistic interconnections among macrolevel political-economic trends, the level of state and institutional policies and practices, and the microlevel of individual experience during immigration and in the subsequent days, months, and years (Willen 2007; Castañeda 2010; Willen, Mulligan, and Castañeda 2011). In doing so, I argue that social and institutional factors must be considered in tandem with the cultural factors known to facilitate the individual behaviors contributing to the Latino Health Paradox.

The Acculturation Concept

The classic definition of acculturation was presented by Redfield, Linton, and Herkovits: "Acculturation comprehends those phenomena which result when groups of individuals having different cultures come into continuous first-hand contact with subsequent changes in the original culture patterns of either or both groups" (1936, 149). This early definition of acculturation emphasizes the role of "culture" as something that is left behind and then learned anew. While it suggests that the interactions among immigrants and community members in their new homes may be bidirectional, this definition describes culture as a somewhat static entity. This general definition has been subsequently amended by scholars of various disciplines in order to allow for a more dynamic understanding of culture and employed to interpret the impact of immigration experiences on health outcomes.

Cross-cultural psychologist John Berry has devoted a great deal of theoretical work to the acculturation concept. Taking what he calls a "rational" approach to understanding acculturation, Berry emphasizes the relationship between cultural context and individual behavioral development. For example, in a seminal article, he poses an important question:

> What happens to individuals, who have developed in one cultural context, when they attempt to live in a new cultural context? If culture is such a powerful shaper of behaviour, do individuals continue to act in the new setting as they did in the previous one, do they change their behavioural repertoire to be more appropriate in the new setting, or is there some complex pattern of continuity and change in how people go about their lives in the new society? (1997, 6)

In asking these questions, Berry (1990, 1997, 1998, 2003) proposes that the powerful psychological dimension of cultural change shapes the ways in which individuals adapt their beliefs and behaviors to fit within a new cultural milieu. Berry suggests that acculturation is the change of the *culture* of a group and the *psychology* of an individual; in this sense, individual experiences do not necessarily conform to those of the cultural group (Berry 1970, 1997). While Berry argues that the most profound changes observed in acculturative encounters occur in the immigrants themselves, there are indeed influences on both host societies and individuals (deemed "acculturating groups"). He believes that there is a general "skeleton" (or "universal qualities") to the aspects of acculturation phenomena and a particular "flesh" evident in specific case studies (1997, 26). For example, variations can be attributed to the individuals' voluntariness to immigrate, ease of mobility, and permanence of settlement in a new location

(Murray and Lopez 1996). Berry often nods to the importance of recognizing national immigration and acculturation policies, ideologies, and attitudes as contributors to the acculturation process, but his research clearly emphasizes the role of "culture" exchange and individual aptitude to the new cultural landscape.

Conversely, anthropological critiques of the acculturation concept address the notion of "culture" itself. For example, Linda Hunt and colleagues (Hunt, Schneider, and Comer 2004) warn that overemphasis on the role of culture and lack of attention to the political-economic and social processes at work in the lives of immigrants can result in cultural stereotyping. In a recent review of the immigration literature, Heide Castañeda argues that considering acculturative experiences as the key contributors to the Latino Health Paradox suggests that "integration into the 'culture' of mainstream society negatively impacts on the health status of immigrants" (2010, 18). Castañeda contends that this argument depends on a number of underlying assumptions, which I present in turn. First, if culture is a key contributor to the health advantage of immigrants, then immigrants migrate to the United States with a collection of "cultural" features or habits that predispose them to better health status (Hunt, Schneider, and Comer 2004). This begs the question: which and whose "cultural" features do new immigrants take up, particularly in a society as diverse as the United States? Second, this argument suggests that cultures are static entities that are not necessarily transformed by the immigrants who move into them. To uphold this argument, then, one would need to assume that the "culture" of Chicago is not only static but also homogenous. Third, because many of these studies are outcomes-focused, they fail to explore mitigating factors such as poor access to health care as a result of cost, location, and access to transportation (Cristancho et al. 2008; Castañeda 2010). And, finally, these studies of acculturation often overlook information about health status over the life course and in different environments. While some studies are beginning to look at the influence of premigration stressors and living conditions (see Himmelgreen et al. 2007), few focus on the ways in which social conditions and personal histories may figure into the relationship between immigration and health. Thus, a focus on culture as the key contributor to health inequities takes away from the powerful role of social determinants on immigrant health (Hirsch 2003b). More specifically, these critiques highlight a seminal argument that gets to the heart of critical medical anthropology: cultural explanations can overshadow the important ways in which political-economic and social inequalities contribute to the unequal distribution of disease among the poor (Mullings 1987; Morsy 1996; Farmer 1999; Singer 2004a).

In chapter 3 I argued that a focus on folk illnesses (or emotions) in diabetes research can overshadow the role played by social forces in the unequal distribution of chronic disease in the United States. In this chapter, I extend that argument by arguing that an overemphasis on "culture" as the root of behavioral change similarly overlooks fundamental social and political-economic processes. For example, cultural factors might play a role in immigrant women's ability to integrate socially, find a job, or access health care, and conversely, structural factors associated with being an immigrant can undermine other forms of social and cultural capital, such as the availability of extended family networks. Thus, we must consider how social and cultural factors jointly contribute to the dual burden of depression and diabetes among immigrants.

At the Border: Mari's Story

A fiercely independent and resilient woman who immigrated alone from Zacatecas to Chicago, Mari participated in a formal interview in 2007 as a part of my exploratory ethnographic research.[1] At that time she was at the clinic with her daughter and a friend, and I heard her laugh resonate across the clinic before we met. When I saw her again at the clinic in 2010, she had lost some weight but looked more haggard than before. She was alone this time and her demeanor had changed: she was more docile, more solemn. While she had insisted on speaking English three years before, Mari only used a few English words during this interview, moving back to Spanish as we discussed some of her more difficult memories. The two narratives did not differ chronologically, but the one presented here, collected in 2010, was more detailed and comprehensive.

One month shy of forty years of age, Mari shared with me a harrowing narrative:

> [I left Mexico] because I needed to work. I needed to look for something else and my friend told me if I come here I'd make a lot of money [pause] so I came and tried it. The first time I came I was sixteen, by myself. [It was] really difficult because I didn't have any money to pay [the *coyotes* to cross the border]. I had to pay with my body. You understand? So it's hard because, I don't know, it's the truth. The guy told me, if you want to go to the United States you have to sleep with me. I didn't have any money to buy food. I didn't have family there, so I said okay.
>
> [I came through] Tijuana. So, I didn't have any family there. No money, no place to live, so I wanted to come here and the guy told me, if you want to go to United States you are sleeping with me. And I didn't have a choice. I had to. [I did that for] three months. I had to do it in Mexico first and then when he took me to Santa Ana, California, I had to stay with him three months to pay [off my debt].
>
> And it's hard. It's hard to make a decision in five seconds, five minutes. It's something like you have to think if you want to leave or you want to stay. I don't know where because I didn't have a place to stay in Tijuana, so he told me if

you're sleeping with me I'll take you to Santa Ana and you [can] stay with my sister in her home and then you look for jobs and that's it. So it was hard for me, you know.

And he took me to Santa Ana and I stayed there with his sister. And I stayed like almost five months in there but I had to clean, cook, take care of the babies and then they wouldn't give me anything. Only food and the house, so when I decided to leave I did it real quick and I came here [to Chicago] with another person. Too many persons you know, different families living together and they do the same job: bring the people from Mexico to here. So, I met a guy and then a lady, and they told me if you want to go to Chicago he'd give me the money and I'd have to give the money back, for Greyhound and then he told me he'd help me to get a job here.

So that's not true. When I [arrived to Chicago] he told the whole family that he was my boyfriend. So I didn't know. I didn't have any family, no friends, no nothing so I stayed with him. I stayed with him for five years. He didn't let me get friends. He closed my door with a lock. I was sixteen. He was thirty-five. So I didn't know what to do. I was scared. I didn't know the people here [in Chicago]. I didn't know nothing. So I stayed with him for five years.

I never really tried to escape. I tried to get a job and he wouldn't let me go. He'd tell me: you can't go nowhere. You have to stay here. He took my shoes. He took my clothes. He put a lock on my door so I didn't know nothing. [pause] Sometimes I would cry and scream, and I would sleep a lot. You know my weight was 305 because I had too much stress. I [felt] scared. I was thinking about my family, and crying for my mom and my dad, for everybody, you know. I missed my family. I remember the first Christmas, when I was in my country, all my family came to my house and made it—you know, dinner. Everything. And then I remember this day by myself in the corner. I don't have nothing to eat and I am thinking about my family. Everything.

When I asked her if she regretted immigrating to the United States, she said that she didn't. However, when I repeated the question differently in Spanish ("Do you ever think it would have been better if you had never left Mexico?"), she replied:

Sometimes. Sometimes, I think its better if I'd stayed with my family, no matter what happens but it's [too] late because I'm here. So I stayed with him and I talked with him about, you know, I want to stay with you. Don't lock my door. I won't go anywhere. Let me talk to the people. You know, let me go out, outside. I want to see the birds, sun, everything. I talked to him and then he let me stay. He took the lock off the door and started talking to the other persons and he changed a little bit. He took me to the store, he bought me food, he gave me everything [. . .].

Some lady tell me that he's like abused me because I am sixteen and he's thirty-five. You know what happens when the guys do that with young people? [pause]

This is abuse. So I told him. If you lock my door and continue like that I [will] call the police. [pause] And he said, no please don't call the police. I will leave your door open. You can go somewhere. You can go to the store. If you want to meet the other ladies in here you can. And it [got] better for me. So I started to take care of babies, got money for myself, and then he changed. Not a lot, but he [began to] leave my door open. I talked to the other ladies, you know. And it was different [. . .].

In like one year probably [I gained] forty pounds. A lot of weight. When I stayed with him my weight was 305. Because I was not walking, doing anything. [I'd] just clean my room, a small room. Not a big room. Cook, clean, eat, and go to sleep. When I got out he'd bring the car to the stairs and the only walking is like three minutes, two minutes a week. It's not enough. That's why. I think that's why I get diabetes. You know my family's got diabetes so it's more risky.

Mari stayed with this man for three more years after he had locked her in his home. I asked her why she felt she had to stay with him. She replied, "Because it's the only person that I got. [pause] The only person [I knew] and I stayed like two years [with him] so I felt like a little, not exactly like love but something like that, you know?" I asked her, "Like you owed him something?" Mari continued:

Something like that. So I stayed with him—for three more years and then he went back to Mexico and he stayed there. So I was free, I was free. But when he left me, I didn't know how to take the bus for work. I didn't know anything. I spoke English a little bit but not enough. So I started looking for a job and working and living by myself, paid my rent, my bills. My life has changed. So it's hard you know? I think that's why I get diabetes.

Once this man left Chicago, Mari began seeking care within the safety-net health system, which is where she was diagnosed with diabetes and continued to receive routine diabetes care nearly two decades later. She also got married and had a daughter. In 2007 Mari had described a positive homelife. In 2010, convinced that her husband was having an affair, she felt less comfortable in her home and neighborhood at large:

The street affects me a great deal because if you go into the street, there are the gangsters. And then when you are walking in the street you feel nervous and angry about all of it. The blacks ask you for a cigarette. They are always asking for everything, and they say to you that you have to give them a cigarette, and it makes me so angry. They begin to fight and it makes me nervous; it makes me sweat and tremble [. . .] It does influence me because it makes my sugar spike. I begin to feel my mouth become dry and I begin trembling. I can't stop trembling for an hour. I think that this influences me a great deal.

While many first-generation immigrant women settle in the Mexican "Mecca" of Chicago (such as Pilsen), Mari's experiences in a mixed ethnic neighborhood southwest of the hospital that is known for its gang violence, food deserts, and poorer health outcomes were major contributors to her stress. Such stress compounded negative feelings surrounding distressing memories of her past that she identified as casual factors in her depression and diabetes. At the time of the interview, Mari had PTSD and moderately severe depression.[2] Even though she had lost more than forty pounds since her captivity two decades previously, at the age of forty Mari already suffered from severe obesity and very poorly controlled diabetes. Mari stated that diabetes had a huge impact on her life, causing her a great deal of worry, fear, and distress.

Immigration, Integration, and Isolation

Understanding immigrant health must occur at the macro-, meso-, and microlevels, as structural, political, and social factors shape individual immigration experiences (Willen 2007). At its most basic level, the decision to migrate from Mexico to the United States expresses an extreme marginalization within the global economy (Castañeda 2010). Immigrants face structural conditions that promote undocumented immigration and produce violence, subjugation, and exploitation both during the migration itself and in the months and years after settling in the new country (DeGenova and Peutz 2010). For example, when Mari used her body as payment for a secure passage across the border, the transaction, and resultant emotional and sexual abuse, stemmed from a desire for financial security in the United States. Such desire cannot be divorced from structural violence and the longstanding myth linking *el norte* (the United States) with prosperity, nor from the United States' impact on economic conditions in Mexico. Nor can it be detached from the severe psychiatric distress related to prolonged symbolic and sexual violence and emotional manipulation and from the poor eating behaviors, activity patterns, and obesity that resulted from it.

While such desire for economic security is well understood within the American imagination, selling one's body for sex and living in captivity upon arrival to the United States do not figure in national interpretations of immigration at large. Rarely do people in the United States hear stories like Mari's, as these individuals often remain hidden, their narratives absent from legal and social discourse: as Paul Farmer suggests, "The suffering of those who are distanced, whether by geography, gender, 'race,' or culture, is sometimes less affecting" on the public than the suffering of individuals whose lives and struggles recall our own (1997, 272). Indeed, some scholars who investigate immigrant health have marginalized such experiences from their interpretations, as well.

Certainly narratives like Mari's are not the norm. Yet, thirteen of the eighteen women who reported immigration stress described it as concurrent with some form of interpersonal abuse: women cited domestic violence in Mexico (as an impetus for immigration), rape while crossing the border, and prolonged interpersonal abuse upon arrival to the United States.[3] Like Mari, many of these are stories of social isolation and marginalization due to undocumented status that cannot be dissociated from immigration policies that criminalize Mexican immigrants. It may be that the staunchly anti-immigrant U.S. agenda that bears, according to De Genova (2005, 62), "the particular imprint of a distinctly anti-Mexican racism,"[4] deters immigrants from helping each other. Being undocumented themselves, family members and neighbors fail to respond to domestic disputes and other instances of abuse, contributing to the lack of social protection for women within the home and of legal protection outside of it. This finding, by highlighting the constraints faced by unauthorized immigration, might contradict other scholarly work that indicates that Mexican immigrant women in the United States hold more agency when compared to women in Mexico (see Hirsch 2003a). On the other hand, Mari's narrative demonstrates how power may lie in a responsive police system: threat of calling the police proved to be the vehicle for Mari to speak truth to power and transform her domestic circumstance.

I see the lack of social protection and the prevailing thread of social isolation to be central to the Latino Health Paradox. While most women's experiences of social isolation were less extreme than Mari's, feelings of liminality as a result of immigration and isolation were salient in their everyday lives. Discussing assimilation into U.S. society, De Genova observes, "Depicted as straddling 'two worlds,' effectively 'displaced,' and existentially homeless, the figure of the immigrant is often characterized by divided desires and a fragmented self. In short, it is always plausible that the immigrant may resist the social forces working to incorporate (and subordinate) his or her difference" (2005, 82). In this sense, the immigration experience itself might contribute to a propensity to socially isolate from others. Indeed, the struggles associated with social integration in Chicago and the longing for a previous time when they were surrounded by parents, siblings, and close friends in Mexico were central to immigrant women's narratives.

This brings forth an important point that was highlighted in chapter 3. Data from Table 3.2 suggest that even though feelings of social isolation are associated with being first-generation immigrants, and such feelings strongly correlate with sexual abuse (Table 3.1), reporting interpersonal abuse strongly correlates with being born in the United States. Congruent with epidemiological studies (Holman, Silver, and Waitzkin 2000; Lown and Vega 2001; Heilemann, Kury, and Lee 2005), Figure 4.1 shows that women born in the United States reported higher rates of interpersonal abuse compared to women born in Mexico.

Just over half of the women born in Mexico (57 percent) reported any exposure to abuse, compared to almost 80 percent of the women born in the United States. The biggest difference was found in the reporting of physical violence. Three-fourths of the women born in the United States reported physical abuse, compared to 43 percent of those born in Mexico. A similar trend characterizes sexual abuse: one in five Mexican-born women reported sexual violence compared to one in three women born in the United States. Thus, these findings indicate that women born in the United States are more likely to report any interpersonal abuse—and physical and sexual abuse specifically—compared to women born in Mexico.

The breakdown of social networks and social protection in which such high rates of abuse appear to be rooted cannot be dissociated from neoliberal economic policies that regulate the exchange of goods and people between Mexico and the United States (Harvey 2005). When asked why there were higher rates of wife battering and child sexual abuse in Chicago compared to rural sending communities in Mexico, many women described a social embeddedness in extended family structures in Mexico that enhanced a sense of family responsibility. In contrast, many women complained of social isolation and lack of family networks upon

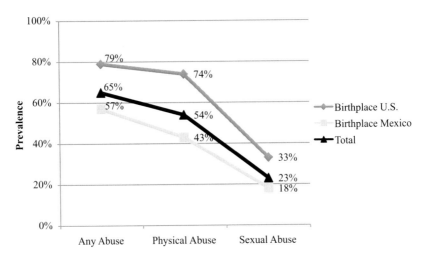

Figure 4.1 Prevalence of interpersonal abuse by birthplace

migration to the United States. In the ever-expanding metropolis of Chicago, many people crowd into small apartments and houses with people who were not necessarily family members. Based on the narrative data, I suggest that changing family structures and moral codes likely contribute to the heightened rates of abuse reported by second-generation women.

Yolanda's story illustrates how the breakdown of moral codes and family networks in the life of a low-income second-generation Mexican immigrant woman might contribute to depression and diabetes in adulthood. Yolanda was a forty-year-old woman whose diabetes care at the GMC was secondary to treatment for severe mental illness. Growing up in Little Village in the 1970s, Yolanda's mother was a heroin addict who often had drug dealers and drug-abusing boyfriends in her home. In addition to her mother's beatings, Yolanda said, "I was also sexually abused by her boyfriends" beginning at the age of five and continuing until she was fourteen years of age, when she moved to her father's residence. As the eldest of three, Yolanda said, stoic and defiant, that she took the abuse to protect her younger siblings.[5] She recalled spending hours of her childhood staring out the window and much of her adolescence and adulthood abusing alcohol and other drugs. She also linked these experiences with her severe depression, which caused extreme weight fluctuations. When she was diagnosed with diabetes, Yolanda explained, "I was 180 [pounds]. I had gained a lot of weight [pause] due to depression. I ate a lot and I stopped just going to places. [pause] Stopped moving around." At the time of the interview Yolanda weighed 124 pounds and had her diabetes well controlled; she mentioned that in recent days she rarely felt like eating. She reported extreme PTSD and depression.[6]

Yolanda's story exemplifies how a breakdown of social protection might affect the lives of children of immigrants who are abandoned by the close networks often characterized as "protective" within Mexican immigrant communities (Eschbach et al. 2004). In addition, neighborhood characteristics such as the lack of affordable housing, economic opportunities, and multigenerational and interfamilial households can contribute to increased stress within low-income Latino populations in U.S. urban centers (Clark et al. 2009). The stress stemming from feeling unsafe or scared by violence within one's physical surroundings was measured by the narrative theme "neighborhood violence" and was more frequently reported by women who were second-generation Mexican Americans, English-speaking, and identified with more "U.S.-oriented values" (see Table 3.2 and Figure 4.2). In some cases stressors such as gang violence and drug abuse were reported in conjunction with related forms of severe distress, such as random shootings and the loss of a child to crossfire.

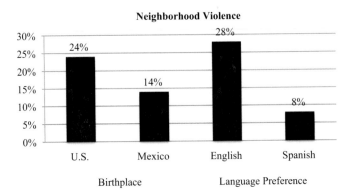

Figure 4.2   Prevalence of neighborhood violence by birthplace and language

The fact that Mexican immigrant women who had settled in the predominantly Mexican neighborhoods of Pilsen and Little Village less frequently reported neighborhood violence may exemplify the protective "barrio" effect, wherein Mexican enclaves have reportedly lower rates of overall street crime, more social cohesion, and more institutional support (Sampson, Morenoff, and Gannon-Rowley 2002; Eschbach et al. 2004; Morenoff, Sampson, and Raudenbush 2006). Hence, the social stresses associated with the political, economic, and social disintegration of the Mexican social networks and community fabric may be at the root of the Latino Health Paradox.

In conclusion, Mari's and Yolanda's experiences illustrate how the intricacies of immigration policy and the lingering effects of social isolation manifest themselves in individual experience. The rising occurrence of interpersonal violence, lack of legal and social protection, and social detachment in the lives of first- and second-generation Mexican immigrant women play a fundamental role in the growing rates of chronic depression and diabetes among them, and indeed in the paradox of health deterioration within U.S. urban spaces.

5

❦

NARRATIVE TO MECHANISM: UNDERSTANDING DISTRESS AND DIABETES

Merrill Singer contends that the syndemics framework requires that we explore the "dynamic relationship involving two or more epidemic diseases or other disorders and the socioenvironmental context that promotes their interaction" (2009a, 29). Heretofore, I have focused a great deal on the contextual and social factors that function as major contributors to the escalating rates of depression and diabetes among first- and second-generation Mexican immigrant women in Chicago. Specifically, I used the extensive narratives of Domenga, Rosie, Marcía, and Mari to elucidate how macrolevel forces, such as poverty and immigration policy, might become transduced into the microlevel stresses experienced in everyday life. Yet, little attention has been directed thus far to the various mechanisms through which social distress might interact with the psychological and physiological domains. Understanding this interaction is essential to VIDDA Syndemic theory, as disease clustering, in the case of depression and diabetes, moves beyond social and emotional aspects. Indeed, evidence suggests that the two diseases are linked biologically.

In this chapter I begin to unpack those interconnections, focusing on research surrounding the synergies between social, psychological, and biological stress. After describing the emergence of diabetes and the behavioral and biological pathways that facilitate its onset, I discuss the impact of stressful experiences on the psychological distress reported by women in my sample. I then discuss in depth six pathways through which diabetes and depression interact and consider social, behavioral, psychological, and biological factors that foster the bidirectional relationship between the two diseases. Finally, I present a VIDDA Syndemic Model and consider the broader implications of VIDDA Syndemic synergies.

The Emergence of Diabetes

Evolutionary theory suggests that the discordance between Paleolithic human genetic make-up and modern lifestyle is a major force behind the diabetes pandemic (Lieberman 2003). Anthropologists explain that Paleolithic humans were well suited for nomadic lifestyles characterized by low-fat diets and frequent physical activity (Eaton, Shostak, and Konner 1988). Changes associated with the agricultural revolution (when people left nomadic life for agricultural settlements) and energized by cultural processes linked more recently with modernization—such as urbanization, westernization of lifestyles, and economic development—have caused modifications in both human diets and physical activity patterns (Eaton, Eaton, and Cordain 2002). For instance, before humans began producing rather than gathering foods, the edible components of grasses were consumed only rarely and in small quantities; today they comprise more than half of the calories and protein consumed by humans worldwide (Cordain 1999). In addition, the reduction of physical activity associated with the more sedentary lifestyles brought about by modernization has had a profound effect on our bodies (Leonard 2001). These behavioral changes have been a driving force behind the rapid increase in obesity and type 2 diabetes rates.

The thrifty genotype hypothesis also raises the possibility of a strong genetic explanation for the high prevalence of obesity and type 2 diabetes. Fifty years ago, geneticist J.V. Neel (1962) proposed that a feast-and-famine existence among American Indian populations had caused a selective advantage and increased reproductive fitness for individuals who could release insulin quickly, thriftily store energy during times of food abundance, and efficiently utilize energy depots during dietary deprivation. Those who accept the thrifty genotype hypothesis argue that modern lifestyles, with their increased food abundance, lack of periodic food shortages, and reduction in energy expenditure, rendered a once adaptive genotype detrimental, leading to obesity and type 2 diabetes (Neel 1962; Neel, Weder, and Julius 1998).

In the early 1990s, David Barker proposed an alternative theory, called the developmental (or "fetal") origins hypothesis, which was critical of the genetic determinism put forth by his predecessors. Barker argued instead that babies who are born small as a result of nutritional stress are more likely to develop chronic diseases later in life when compared to babies with healthier birth weights

(Barker et al. 1989; Barker et al. 1990; Barker 1995, 1999). Based on a number of physiological facts that link low birth weight with adult obesity and diabetes,[1] this theory prioritized social and economic conditions as the root of the unequal distribution of chronic diseases among the population (see Lieberman 2003, 2008; Baker et al. 2008; Ewald 2008; Kuzawa 2008). In the past decade, a number of cohort studies in low- and middle-income countries have confirmed the social origin of prematurity and low-birth weight, stressing the influence of poverty and nutritional stress in utero and during the first years of life (see Norris et al. 2012). In addition, anthropologists have argued that through developmental and epigenetic pathways social influences contribute to the cardiovascular health inequalities found among disadvantaged populations in the United States (Kuzawa and Sweet 2009). Thus, these scholars propose that the high prevalence of diabetes among certain ethnic groups results from political-economic and social conditions, as opposed to a genetic predisposition.

The Biology of Diabetes and Distress

Type 2 diabetes is characterized by insulin resistance. Insulin is produced by the pancreas and largely functions to enable glucose to enter cells where it can be turned into energy. The primary role of insulin is to regulate carbohydrate and fat metabolism by facilitating energy storage in cells; therefore, insulin secretion is closely linked with the concentration of glucose in the blood and is often responsive to eating (Porte, Baskin, and Schwartz 2002). Insulin levels reflect the sensitivity of muscle and adipose tissues to the insulin-mediated transport of glucose into the cells. This sensitivity is determined to a large extent by the total amount of body fat, and particularly by the amount of visceral or abdominal fat, which is more metabolically active than fat located in other parts of the body (Wynne et al. 2005). Normally the body breaks down carbohydrates for energy, but individuals with insulin resistance are unable to reduce blood glucose concentrations to normal levels. Insulin resistance contributes to an increased storage and circulation of excess fat in the abdomen because the body uses these fats for fuel when glucose is unavailable (Epel et al. 2000; Wynne et al. 2005).

Insulin is also closely linked with the brain, as insulin receptors are widely distributed throughout the brain and the hypothalamus in particular. The hypothalamus has both hunger and satiety centers that influence eating behaviors and are associated with a number of neuropeptides and hormones connected with eating and fat storage. Normally, insulin acts through the hypothalamus to decrease food intake and body weight. For example, when insulin causes a reduction in blood glucose levels, it stimulates eating (Wynne et al. 2005). However, when individuals are chronically stressed,[2] the stress hormone cortisol acts on fat cells throughout the body to make them insulin resistant, while at the same time the body releases high levels of glucose (Robinson and Fuller 1985). High levels of cortisol also are linked with eating behaviors, such as increased appetite, sugar cravings, and weight gain (Epel et al. 2001; Wynne et al. 2005), thereby complicating the body's ability to regulate carbohydrate metabolism and increasing fat storage. Thus, chronic stress is physiologically linked with the onset of diabetes.

In addition, a number of culturally and socially mediated behaviors have been found to affect the physiological processes associated with diabetes (Lieberman 2003, 2006, 2008). For example, social contexts, cultural beliefs and practices, interpersonal relationships, and even atmospherics (such as lighting and music) have been linked with eating behaviors (Epel et al. 2001; Turner et al. 2008). In fact, family-level factors, such as ethnicity and cultural habits, have proven to be *stronger* mediators of taste preferences and food choices than biological drives or innate tendencies (Messer 1986; Birch 1987; Simoons 1994; Rozin 1996; Turner et al. 2008). Even more, there is a strong association between the common mental disorders of depression and anxiety and the propensity to gain weight via eating behaviors (Epel et al. 2001). These studies further emphasize the need for a multidimensional understanding of the social, psychological, and cultural factors associated with diabetes.

Distress in the Mind and Body

As I pointed out in chapter 1, all my interlocutors had been diagnosed with type 2 diabetes and presented other markers of psychological and physical distress. Table 5.1 profiles the mental and physical health of these women. The table presents measures of depression and post-traumatic stress disorder, in addition to diabetes control (hemoglobin A1c), obesity (body mass index and waist circumference), and blood pressure (systolic and diastolic). I will discuss these data in turn.

Table 5.1 Psychological and biological stresses (n = 121)

Stress Measure	Mean (+/− Standard Deviation)
Post-Traumatic Stress Disorder (PCL-C)	31.0 (+/− 15.9)
Depression (CES-D)	18.3 (+/− 14.7)
Hemoglobin A1c (percent of HbA1c)	9.05 (+/− 2.12)
Body Mass Index (kg/m²)	35 (+/− 7.6)
Waist Circumference (cm)	43.8 (+/− 6.04)
Systolic Blood Pressure (mm Hg)	146.5 (+/− 21.5)
Diastolic Blood Pressure (mm Hg)	79.8 (+/− 11.0)

Table 5.1 highlights the severe psychological distress reported by approximately half the women in my study and indicates that average measures of post-traumatic stress disorder (PTSD) and depression were slightly higher than traditional cutoff points to signify the disorders. Two in five women reported symptoms of PTSD according to the PTSD Checklist—Civilian Version, with a mean score of 31, which was just higher than an accepted PTSD cutoff point for primary care settings (PCL-C $\geq$ 30) (Walker et al. 2002). These findings reveal very high rates of PTSD when compared to studies that report a PTSD prevalence of 7 percent among the general U.S. population (Dohrenwend et al. 1984), 19 percent among a clinical veteran population up to six months after returning from combat and 9 percent a decade after service (Dohrenwend et al. 2006), and an 8 percent prevalence among veterans with diabetes (Trief et al. 2006).[3] The extremely high PTSD prevalence of 41 percent among the women with diabetes in my study resembled the results found in another clinical sample of Mexican immigrant women seeking primary care in California (not discriminated according to a diabetes diagnosis), which showed a 38 percent prevalence (Heilemann, Kury, and Lee 2005). These findings suggest that the high rate of PTSD may be associated with heightened exposure to stressful or traumatic events and with the fact that those who seek clinical care are more likely to carry psychological distress. The current literature also suggests that women with depression often report high rates of traumatic experience and PTSD symptoms (Breslau et al. 1997; Bromet, Sonnega, and Kessler 1998; Heilemann, Kury, and Lee 2005).

One in every two women I met reported depression according to a modest cutoff point for likely depression measured by the Center for Epidemiologic Studies Depression Scale (CES-D $\geq$ 16); even the mean CES-D score exceeded that point (Table 5.1: CES-D = 18.3). A more rigorous cutoff point (CES-D $\geq$ 24), which suggests that someone "very likely has depression," indicates that one in three women were likely to be depressed. It is not surprising that these women had much higher rates of depression when compared to non-diabetic populations, whose rate is around 8 percent (Gonzalez et al. 2010); yet, these data were notably higher than the 25 percent prevalence of depression found among people with diabetes in clinical populations (Anderson et al. 2001). Nevertheless, compared to the shockingly high rates of interpersonal abuse and the cumulative impact of social distress revealed through the women's life history narratives, we might interpret a 34 percent prevalence of depression to be somewhat modest.

The biomarkers revealed more "objective" measures of stress over the life course. All the women interviewed for this study had type 2 diabetes and more than 90 percent of these women had poorly controlled diabetes according to the American Diabetic Association (ADA: HbA1c $\geq$ 6.5) (Sacks et al. 2011).

The average measure of hemoglobin A1c, an assessment of diabetes control over the past three months, was 9.05 (SD +/– 2.12). Based on these data alone, it is not surprising that the women's bodies were generally pear shaped with a mean waist circumference of 43.8 cm, which is characteristic of those with diabetes, and average body mass index was 35 kg/m², indicating severe obesity. Furthermore, average blood pressure was slightly higher than the level considered "at risk" for elevated blood pressure (BP > 120/80), with a mean systolic blood pressure at 146.5 mm HG and mean diastolic blood pressure at 79.8 mm HG.

Alone, these data reveal striking rates of mental distress and concordant chronic disease. However, to understand the meaning behind and the intersections among these data, further analyses are necessary. The next section examines the interconnections among social, psychological, and biological domains that are intrinsic to the clustering of VIDDA Syndemic interactions.

Cumulative Effects

A large body of literature has shown that early life stresses can increase the risk of psychological and physical disorders as adults (Cohen and Williamson 1988; Boyce and Chesterman 1990; Chrousos and Gold 1992; McEwen 1998; McEwen and Seeman 1999; Sapolsky 2002; McEwen 2004). Boyce and Chesterman (1990) suggest that exposure to numerous negative life events during childhood may result in a physiological change that causes children to have less cardiovascular reactivity when stressed. This effect may have long-term consequences and may be a major contributor to the clustering of diabetes and depression among the Mexican immigrant women in this study.

But how does one measure the link between social suffering and physiology? Seeman and colleagues (2004) propose that disease risk may be measured in terms of allostatic load. Allostatic load is defined as a measure of cumulative impact of adaptive physiological responses that chronically exceed optimal operating ranges and affect the body's regulatory systems. In this sense, allostatic load serves as a mediator between life experiences and biological risk: each stressor increases biological risk for disease, and individuals exposed to a certain number of stressors (such as four or more) may be more likely to have poor health outcomes than others. While this approach certainly may be a way to "measure" social suffering, each stressor must be interpreted carefully because the intensity, duration, and form of each stressor may affect physiology differently. Nevertheless, the notion of allostatic load informs the syndemics approach because it shows how social stressors are inscribed in the body and may be reflected in known burdens of diagnosed disease. Thus, this approach might provide one way to measure the impact of structural violence over an individual's life course.

In Table 5.2 I evaluated the relationship of narratively generated social stresses with psychological distress.[4] The data reveal that interpersonal abuse is independently associated with both depression and PTSD, and that these relationships exist when evaluating physical abuse and sexual abuse independently. Feelings of social isolation, health stress, and diabetes distress also were significantly associated with depression and PTSD. However, salient sources of social distress in women's lives, such as loss of a family member, neighborhood violence, financial insecurity, and work stress were not significant predictors of psychological distress among my interlocutors (Table 5.2). This does not mean that these sources of stress were insignificant (see Table 3.1). Rather it means that within this population diagnosed with diabetes, they were not significant predictors of depression or PTSD.

The strong association between interpersonal abuse and psychiatric distress is not surprising, as there are established links between reporting abuse and

Table 5.2   Unadjusted linear regressions of stressors with psychological distress (n = 121)

Stressors	Depression			PTSD		
	Effect	**95% CI**	**P**	**Effect**	**95% CI**	**P**
Any Abuse	**10.1**	**4.89,15.4**	**0.00**	**14.5**	**9.08,19.9**	**0.00**
Physical Abuse	**8.51**	**3.41,13.6**	**0.00**	**13.2**	**7.92,18.4**	**0.00**
Sexual Abuse	**10.7**	**4.69,16.7**	**0.00**	**13.5**	**7.15,19.9**	**0.00**
Social Isolation	**14**	**7.02,21.1**	**0.00**	**11.1**	**3.29,18.9**	**0.01**
Health Stress	**6.37**	**1.14,11.6**	**0.02**	3.67	−2.07,9.41	0.21
Family Stress	3.59	−1.70,8.87	0.18	2.65	3.07,8.38	0.36
Loss of Family Member	1.74	−3.78,7.26	0.53	3.35	−2.59,9.29	0.27
Financial Stress	3.04	−2.52,8.60	0.28	3.03	−2.98,9.03	0.32
Neighborhood Violence	1.86	−5.16,8.87	0.60	−0.23	−7.81,7.35	0.95
Immigration Stress	−2.47	−9.93,4.99	0.51	−0.84	−8.91,7.23	0.84
Work Stress	2.17	−5.30,9.63	0.57	5.95	−2.04,13.9	0.14
Language	−2.46	−7.77,2.84	0.36	−2.85	−8.58,2.87	0.33
Birthplace	−3.96	−9.50,1.58	0.16	−5.72	−11.7,0.22	0.06
Acculturation	0.77	−0.69,2.23	0.30	**1.58**	**0.03,3.14**	**0.05**
Documented Status	−2.82	−8.77,3.13	0.35	−3.36	−9.78,3.05	0.30
Diabetes Distress	**4.00**	**2.64,5.38**	**0.00**	**2.88**	**1.29,4.47**	**0.00**
Depression	-	-	-	**0.71**	**0.69,0.95**	**0.00**
Cumulative Stress[φ]	**3.51**	**1.87,5.16**	**0.00**	**3.63**	**1.84,5.42**	**0.00**

[φ] Number of Stresses reported in Life History Narratives (0 to 9).

suffering from depression, particularly among those who report sexual abuse (Sciolla et al. 2011). Many women reported the cumulative effects of domestic abuse and sexual violence during childhood, verbal and physical battering within a marriage, and emotional neglect or social isolation in late adulthood. It is critical to recognize that the interaction and effects of two or more stresses on depression may supersede the effects of any one form of stress, as difficult experiences rarely occur in isolation and cumulative effects can significantly increase psychiatric distress (Dong et al. 2004). Finally, we must remember that biological pathways link these cumulative stresses to depression and diabetes, and that these pathways are heightened when one experiences extreme distress during childhood (Felitti et al. 1998; McEwen 2004).

Although it is widely recognized that social integration affects mental health (Berkman et al. 2000), I was surprised to find that feelings of social isolation were the strongest predictor of depression among my interlocutors (Table 5.2). As I described in chapter 3, this narrative theme represents a small number of women, the majority of whom (90 percent) were first-generation Mexican immigrants and communicated a sense of longing for their parents, siblings, and friends in Mexico as well as a feeling of social detachment from their families and social networks in Chicago. Almost all of these women had a history of abuse and many experienced more general family stress. The strong correlation between sexual abuse and feelings of social isolation (Table 3.1) might indicate that women with a history of sexual abuse are more likely to isolate themselves socially, and that those who detach from social networks might be at higher risk for depression (Table 5.2). Understanding these experiences is particularly important because social epidemiologists have found strong associations between social isolation and adverse health generally (Berkman and Syme 1979), and depression among Latino immigrants specifically (Vega et al. 2011). Thus, the examples of social detachment presented in this book exemplify how social realities of interpersonal abuse and immigration might interact with the link between social networks and health.

The connection between interpersonal abuse and depression is a central tenet of VIDDA Syndemic theory and therefore required further evaluation. In Table 5.3 I evaluated the linear relationship of interpersonal abuse with depression, adjusting for feelings of social isolation, health stress, and diabetes distress alone and together.[5] All models in Table 5.3 were also adjusted for age, education, income, language preference, acculturation (ARSMA-II), and body mass index (BMI). These data indicate that reporting of any interpersonal abuse was independently associated with depression (Model 1), and this association was maintained when adjusting for social isolation (Model 2), health stress (Model 3), and diabetes distress (Model 4) alone or together (Model 5).

Table 5.3   Adjusted linear regression models of abuse and depression (n = 121)

	Model 1 Beta (95%CI)	Model 2 Beta (95%CI)	Model 3 Beta (95%CI)	Model 4 Beta (95%CI)	Model 5 Beta (95%CI)
Interpersonal Abuse	10.1*** (4.56–15.7)	7.06* (1.54,12.6)	9.30*** (3.76,14.8)	10.4*** (5.57,15.1)	7.81** (2.88,12.8)
Social Isolation	-	14.2*** (6.52,21.8)	-	-	9.86** (2.96,16.7)
Health Stress	-	-	5.37* (0.11–10.6)	-	2.57 (–1.99,7.12)
Diabetes Distress	-	-	-	4.15*** (2.86,5.45)	3.59*** (2.27,4.91)

$*p < 0.05$; $**p < 0.01$; $***p < 0.001$.

These quantitative findings reveal associations that are central to VIDDA Syndemic synergies, as interpersonal abuse, social isolation, and physical health are fundamental to the social and psychological well-being of the women in my study. However, we must also think critically about these associations and consider what Singer (2004b) has called "oppression illness." This concept brings to light the fact that those who internalize a negative understanding of themselves and the world are more likely to report stressful experiences (Dohrenwend et al. 1984; Watson and Clark 1984). On the one hand, these women may have experienced negative affect as a result of chronic adversity, meaning that they maintained a relatively constant negative state of feeling distressed, nervous, angry, guilty, or scornful (Watson and Clark 1984). On the other hand, individuals who internalize adverse experiences may be prone to develop diabetes as a result of chronic psychological stress. In other words, the high rates of interpersonal abuse, feelings of social isolation, and health stress reported by the women may be biased by their physical condition. While it is impossible to make this claim from my data without a comparative group of people without diabetes, a growing body of research indicates that individuals with depression are at greater risk for the onset of diabetes (Talbot and Nouwen 2000; Musselman et al. 2003; Knol et al. 2006; Golden et al. 2007; Golden et al. 2008; Mezuk et al. 2008).

Diabetes and Depression

A growing body of research substantiates the claim of a bidirectional relationship between depression and diabetes. In this section, I describe in depth two hypotheses that define this relationship: one is that depression causes diabetes and the other is that diabetes causes depression. I present five pathways that have been proposed in the literature to describe how depression may contribute to diabetes onset, including neurohormonal changes, glucose transport, inflammatory activation, behavioral factors, and the use of antidepressants (Golden et al. 2007).[6] In addition, I discuss the widely accepted claim that the severity of diabetes, including the stress of managing the disease and coping with its complications, contributes to depression.

The first pathway linking depression with diabetes involves neurohormonal processes associated with the biological stress response. At its most basic level, when the brain experiences or perceives something to be stressful, it activates corticotropin releasing hormone (CRH) within fifteen seconds of the initial stress response. CRH then triggers the release of hormones within the sympathetic nervous system and hypothalamic-pituitary-adrenal (HPA) axis. The sympathetic nervous system instantaneously releases epinephrine or norepinephrine to initiate a "fight or flight" response, respectively. Working over a period of minutes or hours, the HPA-axis secretes an array of releasing hormones, including cortisol, which begins the extended stress response.[7] Concurrently, stress triggers the pancreas to release glucagon. Together, these hormones raise the levels of sugar in the blood, as they are essential for mobilizing energy during stress. However, increased secretion of CRH as a result of chronic stress antagonizes the hypoglycemic effects of insulin, leading to the insulin resistance characteristic of diabetes (see Musselman et al. 2003; Sapolsky 2004).

The second pathway linking depression with diabetes involves glucose transporters (GLUT), which facilitate the entry of glucose, a necessary metabolic substrate associated with energy, into cells. Within the brain, glucose utilization is an indicator of neuronal activity. However, depressed individuals display decreased glucose utilization in the left lateral prefrontal cortex of the brain (Musselman et al. 2003). Antidepressant treatment has been shown to reverse the alteration in cerebral glucose utilization among those who are depressed (Hurwitz et al. 1990; Martinot et al. 1990), thereby substantiating the physiological link between depression and glucose transport. Scientists also suggest that there are defects in glucose transport across membranes associated with cortisol (Robinson and Fuller 1985). In addition, high concentrations of insulin-sensitive glucose transporter-4 (GLUT4) exist in adipose tissue, muscles, and the heart, and there is evidence of abnormal glycogen synthesis in muscle tissue among people with type 2 diabetes (Petersen and Shulman 2002).

The third pathway indicates that inflammation and the associated secretion of proinflammatory cytokines by activated cells can mediate the association of depression and diabetes (Kiecolt-Glaser and Glaser 2002; Black 2003; Musselman et al. 2003; Ford and Erlinger 2004). Proinflammatory cytokines, including interleukin (IL)-1, IL-6, and tumor necrosis factor-α (TNF-α) can induce a constellation of symptoms characteristic of major depression, including fatigue and reduction in self-care (Musselman et al. 2003). Inflammatory changes linked with IL-6 have been found to result from stress hormones, and IL-6 specifically can be found in people with depression. Fat cells are an important source of cytokines, including interleukin 6 (IL-6) and C-reactive protein (CRP), which play a dominant role in the inflammatory processes via visceral fat deposits and are associated with obesity, hypertension, increased blood pressure, and insulin resistance (Black 2003; Musselman et al. 2003; Dandona, Aljada, and Bandyopadhyay 2004). Because IL-6 is capable of crossing the blood-brain barrier, interacting with processes within the hypothalamus, there may be biological interactions where diabetes functions as a contributor to depression, as well.

The fourth pathway is well established and addresses how depression may have a negative impact on healthy behaviors, such as dietary intake, physical activity, medication adherence, and smoking, which may increase the risk of developing diabetes (Musselman et al. 2003; Golden et al. 2007). In a study of the bidirectional relationship of diabetes and depression in a multiethnic sample, Sherita Hill Golden and colleagues (2008) found that individuals with more depression symptoms often reported behaviors associated with diabetes risk. Their findings correspond with prior studies showing that those suffering from depression tend to be female, to consume higher caloric diets, to be less physically active, to smoke, and to have a lower income (Carnethon et al. 2003; Arroyo et al. 2004; Everson-Rose et al. 2004; Golden et al. 2007; Golden et al. 2008). However, adjusting for these factors did not significantly affect the relationship between diabetes and depression, suggesting that they do not fully explain the relationship between the two diseases (Golden et al. 2008).

Many of my interlocutors identified chronic stress and psychological distress as major contributors to behaviors linked with obesity, including increased consumption of higher caloric diets and reduced activity patterns. For example, some women described "stuffing" negative emotions with comfort foods, and many identified negative emotions as contributors to diabetes onset through stress-induced eating. For example, Rosie stated, "My stress level was very, very high and I compensated by eating whatever I wanted at any time I wanted. So, the factors to get diabetes are family, stress, and bad eating habits. [pause] Very bad eating habits." Similarly, Mari's narrative demonstrates how negative feelings, in addition to her extreme circumstances, facilitated poor dietary and exercise patterns that contributed to the tremendous weight gain that led to diabetes onset.

At the same time, a number of women connected poor eating patterns with negative emotions resulting from specific stresses, from financial insecurity to family problems and memories of childhood abuse. Ramona, a forty-year old woman who grew up in Chicago and was sexually abused by her father, said:

> I think that's why I put on this weight too, because he always used to talk about, he'd just say, "You never gonna find a husband—nobody wants a fat ass." Just things like that, he would just throw at me. I think that's why I put the weight on—'cause I didn't want him touching me [. . .] I remember when I was in grade school, the highest I was I remember being a size 12. Then through high school I was a size 18 to 24. Then after that, I just [pause] I lost the weight and then I just went from 24 again. It's just like, I missed the in-between—I don't remember even being size 20, 22, just 18 to 24, from 24 to 32. And the biggest I was is 36. [pause] And right now I'm like a size 30 [. . .] I'm just an emotional eater, I guess that's what they call it.

A fifth pathway shows how weight gain and obesity that result from using antidepressant medication may predispose depressed individuals to diabetes (Golden et al. 2007). Although rarely described in women's life stories, weight gain is relatively common during both acute and long-term treatment with antidepressants (Nihalani et al. 2011). Significant weight gain during treatment for acute depression or weight gain that continues despite achieving full remission of depressive symptoms are likely to be side effects of antidepressant treatment (Fava 2000). Specifically, beta-3 adrenergic receptors found in adipose tissue play an active role in weight control by converting fat into energy, especially in response to stress hormones; psychotropics with higher affinities for these receptors are strongly correlated with weight gain, while others are not (Strosberg and Pietri-Rouxel 1996). Even more, a depressed state increases the likelihood of excessive eating and reduced physical activity, which further increases one's risk for weight gain and insulin resistance. A negative feedback loop, then, contributes to a lower probability that overweight and obese people will exercise.

Finally, a large body of research has explored how diabetes itself increases the possibility of depression. A meta-analysis concluded that people with diabetes are twice as likely to be depressed as people without diabetes (Anderson et al. 2001). While such a finding might suggest that those with depression are more susceptible to diabetes, it should also be noted that diabetes is a profoundly distressing disease. Diabetes management requires dedication to taking medicines at the same time each day, eating healthy and diverse foods, and exercising regularly. Many patients struggle to meet these requirements because the behavioral and dietary changes mandated by doctors run up against cultural norms and environmental limitations, including the hindrances of having to eat special foods apart from the family and not feeling safe enough to walk in one's neighborhood alone. Moreover, disadvantaged populations are more likely to experience diabetes complications—such as nephropathy, retinopathy, neuropathy, macrovascular disease, and amputations—as a result of living in resource-poor settings and receiving delayed care. Thus, multiple behavioral and physical changes experienced as a result of living with diabetes may affect the mental health of diabetes patients, especially as the disease progresses and in case of individuals with poor access to health care.

Towards a VIDDA Syndemic Framework

Singer describes the syndemics framework as inherently multidimensional. In this chapter I have attempted to outline what biological processes underscore VIDDA interactions by highlighting the mechanisms through which biological stress may contribute to insulin resistance. Genetics, biology, health behaviors, and obesity are fundamental to diabetes incidence and the most commonly recognized variables in biomedicine and public health. I argue, however, that it is the macrolevel political-economic processes and microlevel social stressors that contribute to the much higher rates of depression and diabetes among low-income Mexican immigrants when compared to the general population. Thus, we must understand these epidemic health problems to reflect epidemic social problems revealed through the life stories of the women I met.

I have developed a framework to illustrate how structural *violence, immigration-*related stress, *depression, diabetes*, and interpersonal *abuse*, which are experienced as a single multifaceted force, together contribute to poorer health among Mexican immigrant women in Chicago. Figure 5.1 shows the various elements of the VIDDA Syndemic that I have deconstructed throughout this book, and situates them within a broader context of confluent factors in order to demonstrate the complexities that shape Mexican immigrant women's health and social well-being in Chicago.

The point of this figure is to reinforce the notion that a syndemic is not an "end point." Rather it is a synergy of diverse factors that come together to shape epidemic health and social problems. The centrifugal interactions among structural, social, psychological, and biological processes in the VIDDA Syndemic converge to cultivate experiences such as those narrated in this book, and collectively contribute to the disease and suffering expressed by my interlocutors. Structural dimensions mediate Mexican immigrant women's extremely high incidence of diabetes and depression, from the foods they put into their bodies to the care they might seek to alleviate mental distress. Sociocultural processes such as the structure of power and agency associated with gender and

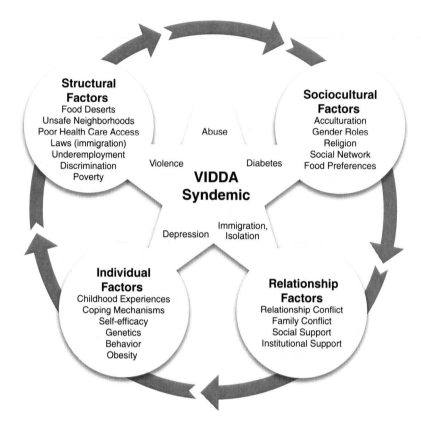

Figure 5.1 The VIDDA Syndemic Model[8]

ethnicity can shape how each woman perceives and responds to experiences of
trauma and subjugation, and these responses can have psychological and biological consequences. Concurrently, interpersonal relationships play a critical role in
each woman's ability to endure life's hardships and enjoy its blessings. Individual
life experiences in addition to individual-level responses to life's challenges are
intrinsic to the embodiment and experience of VIDDA. Thus, the VIDDA
Syndemic introduces an integrated analysis of how political-economic and social
conditions that facilitate stressful experiences can be synergistically tied to the
biological mechanisms linking depression and diabetes that I have outlined in
this chapter. *Narrative to mechanism*, these adverse conditions come together to
create the VIDDA Syndemic.

CONCLUSION

In the introduction, I explained that the syndemics orientation departs from traditional biomedical approaches that treat disease as a distinct entity, detached from social contexts (Singer and Clair 2003). Examining the problem of diabetes as a singular disease is limiting, because it requires us to overlook the fundamental links between diabetes and the macrolevel forces that facilitate its clustering among the poor. As Singer comments, "a fundamental aspect of the syndemic perspective is its focus on the reasons threats to health tend to congregate in particular populations at particular points in time and place" (2009a, 134). The VIDDA Syndemic describes an interactive framework through which the social and epidemiological significance of diabetes cannot be understood apart from the clustering of depression and adverse social conditions. At the same time, the emergence of the VIDDA Syndemic in Chicago cannot be dissociated from the current great inequities of both wealth and health within the city. Nor can it be dissociated from the structural inequalities that over the past thirty years have facilitated the syndemic emergence.

Throughout this book I have presented numerous life stories of women who personify the complexity of these syndemic interactions, revealing interconnections of childhood trauma and unabated depression, immigration and sexual coercion, sexual violence and traumatic memory, immigration and struggle for social integration, family stress and neighborhood discord, depression and social isolation, and the everyday stress of managing diabetes. These stresses facilitate individualized behaviors, such as overeating, internalizing emotion, and lacking physical activity, and increase rates of chronic depression and the associated diabetes risks and complications. The "self" emerging from these lived experiences cannot be separated from the larger political-economic context, as structural and symbolic forms of violence contribute to shaping individual ways of being in the world. Interpersonal abuse, in particular, is one important manifestation of political-economic and social realities that cannot be understood apart from the emotional forces that contribute to depression and diabetes. Even more, the individual experience of Mexican immigrants in Chicago must be seen as part of a larger political system that often associates immigration with illegality, feeding discrimination, and threats of deportation. Traumatic border crossings and lack of social protection upon arrival to Chicago also cause extreme distress and insecurity.

By recognizing that depression functions as a precipitator of diabetes, we must also recognize that diabetes is one of multiple stressful factors contributing to depression, particularly among the socially disadvantaged in the United States (Osborn et al. 2010). In Singer's terminology, diabetes and depression constitute a bidirectional syndemic among Mexican women in Chicago, in that each of these diseases adversely impacts the other (2009a). This is a critical point because too often depression is understood to be a byproduct of disease and treated pharmacologically with an emphasis on disease-related factors. By contrast, social and psychological factors should be understood as part of a negative feedback loop, as social and emotional distresses contribute to depression, which thereby contributes to the onset and complications of diabetes, which then loops back to cause further negative social and psychological consequences.

In this conclusion I discuss one final story to comment on the essential role of integrative health care in mitigating the devastating effects of the VIDDA Syndemic. I use Teresa's narrative to address three questions posed by Merrill Singer in the conclusion of his landmark book, *An Introduction to Syndemics* (2009a), concerning the role of biomedicine in the treatment and care of syndemics. Indeed, in the United States there is a legacy of marginalizing social and emotional factors within the culture of biomedicine (Good 1994) and in the practice of social and mental health services within safety-net health care (Wilkinson and Pickett 2009). In doing so, I wish to emphasize the importance of the institutional dimension of the VIDDA Syndemic.

Seeking Support

Teresa sat alone in the waiting room of the GMC as she awaited a routine diabetes appointment, engrossed in the newest Spanish-language issue of *People*. Teresa was a fifty-one-year-old mother of three who emigrated from a small town in Mexico. As the eldest of six children, Teresa attended limited schooling and spent much of her childhood raising her siblings. At sixteen Teresa left her mother and siblings in Mexico to join her father in Chicago. Two years later she married a Mexican immigrant she met in Chicago who was, like her, disinterested in childbearing. After spending much of her childhood caring for children, Teresa was seeking independence. Nevertheless, within months she was pregnant. Teresa said that for a woman who never anticipated having a child of her own, bearing three children in three years was difficult. At last her third child was a boy, and her husband was satisfied. These children are at the center of her life story.

Teresa's story is a somewhat typical case. When she arrived to Chicago thirty-six years ago, Teresa longed for her mother in Mexico and felt that her social and emotional life was at the juncture of Mexico and Chicago. For many years Teresa endured alcoholism and the resultant verbal abuse and emotional manipulation from her husband. She attributed the abuse to her husband's genuine feelings of insecurity due to the fact that she was a more effective wage earner, working as a payroll supervisor for a center for the elderly. Scholars link such feelings with modernity and the shifting balance of gender and power within Mexican marriages (Hirsch 2003a). At the same time, the well-being of her children and grandchildren had come to consume Teresa's everyday life. Importantly, much of her narrative and life story at large revolved around ongoing family discord and fear for her children's safety. Teresa was particularly fearful that her children were participating in gangs and using drugs.

Teresa was a very confident, forthright woman who did not report any severely traumatic experiences or PTSD. At the time of the interview, Teresa reported minimal depression but stated that she had experienced depression in the past. She associated much of her emotion with family problems, and many of these concerns were other people's tribulations that she took on as her own. Indeed, she felt the suffering of others quite deeply. For example, as many Mexicans do (Poss and Jezewski 2002), Teresa linked her diabetes onset with a frightful experience (susto) associated with the discovery that her brother's child was not his own, and that his wife had been unfaithful for many years. This family discovery, and the ongoing support for her brother, continued to be a major stress in her life. In this way, Teresa's family's problems were at the center of her life and must be understood to be integral to her mental health and diabetes self-care. Interestingly, despite her relatively stable mental health, Teresa's diabetes was poorly controlled (HbA1c:9.4).

Teresa explained, "Last time I came to Cook County I brought with me four problems." She sat relaxed against the back of her chair, with one hand on the table, and the other in her purse sitting in the chair next to her. She continued:

> I felt very bad. One [problem was] because my son's wife left him in September for Mexico because their son was using drugs and was in gangs. The other problem

was with the other son, that his wife went to Mexico with their children [. . .] Later there were other problems with my brother-in-law, because his wife had children with another man [. . .] Then he came to my house, and talked about all of those problems, the whole history. And the fourth problem was with my daughter's boyfriend. I went to ask the guy if he was going to stay with her and he said, "whatever she decides." This was the fourth thing that happened when I arrived here in pain, with my sugar so high. I was feeling really bad and said to [my primary care doctor] that I wanted to kill that fourth person [the daughter's boyfriend].

They brought me to the psychiatrist. They brought me a doctor to talk with, and then the doctor asks me, "So what happened?" I spoke with him about my problems. He said, "You don't have any problems." Then he prescribed me Prozac— the pill. For three months.[1]

[The medication] helped me. But I went on speaking with God and do you know what God told me? I am not going to depend on a drug to feel better. I am going to go on without a drug and until now I have not had to return to the medicines. I have heard that they are very addictive and I didn't take them for more than three months. But in my mind I began to think that they weren't my problems, that everyone has their own problems. That this is what I am trying to understand within the Mexican culture. That this is what you look at in our family, taking on too many other people's problems. For this I said that emotionally diabetes forms as part of our life.

Treatment for the VIDDA Syndemic

Teresa's story brings forth three critical questions integral to mitigating the effects of the VIDDA Syndemic, as posed by Singer (2009a, 206). First, what can biomedicine do to address the social causes of syndemics? Second, for patients who are suffering from multiple interacting diseases, what is the best course of medical treatment? Can entwined syndemic diseases be treated simultaneously? Third, how can biomedicine avoid syndemic interactions that worsen as a result of medical treatment?

The first question attends to the inherently social aspect of syndemics, which is evident in the women's narratives and must be addressed in medical care and treatment. Like Teresa, many women expressed that discord from their social lives was intrinsic to their well-being. When Teresa came to seek diabetes care at the clinic, she brought along four problems, all of which were the conflicts of others. In this way, Teresa indicated that her social world could not be dissociated from her diabetes care. This finding suggests that clinicians must address the social and psychological dimensions of their patients' lives in order to understand and effectively communicate with their patients about diabetes management (Loewe and Freeman 2000).

Yet, traditional biomedicine has been slow to realize that social factors play an important role in disease (Good 1994; Farmer et al. 2006; Singer 2009a). This is exemplified in the actions of her primary care physician who, despite Teresa's understanding that her social life was affecting her diabetes, connected her with a psychiatrist to address her problems. This action might be interpreted as a belief common among biomedical doctors that structural and social interventions are "not our job" (Farmer et al. 2006). Similarly, Teresa felt largely dismissed and dismayed when the psychiatrist prescribed a medication that she did not believe she needed, rather than providing an opportunity for her to discuss her problems. On the one hand, the perceived dismissal of Teresa's problems might lie in part in a greater inability of primary care settings to take notice of social stresses, because much of the attention is devoted to the physical problems associated with diabetes (Weiner et al. 2007, 2010). On the other hand, part of the perceived dismissal of Teresa's social and psychological needs might be attributed to the fact that institutional demands often constrain clinicians' time and prevent the in-depth dialogue necessary to understand the patients' social and emotional problems.

The second question brings forth the issue of medical treatment, including the potential effect of treating diabetes and depression simultaneously. Teresa's narrative exemplifies how medicating social and psychological problems, as opposed to addressing their roots, fails to deal with them in the clinical sphere. Additionally, it is interesting that even though there is evidence that family discord plays a powerful role in diabetes management among Latinos (Fisher et al. 2000), clinicians rarely attend to family conflict and stress in clinical care. The consequence of dismissing Teresa's social and emotional problems in her medical care is evident in her poorly controlled diabetes.

Thus, there is an obvious need for treatments that address the negative feedback loop between structural and social problems, depression, and diabetes. There is precedence for this approach, but often clinicians who practice holistic, integrative primary care and social medicine are considered to be somewhat radical. Perhaps the most famous current model of this kind was designed by Partners in Health (PIH), an organization cofounded by medical anthropologists and physicians Paul Farmer and Jim Yong Kim (Farmer et al. 2001). This model recognizes that addressing structural and social problems is central to mitigating the effects of structural violence and improving community health. Their projects in Boston, as well as in Peru, Rwanda, Russia, and Haiti, have proven successful in improving the health of extremely poor communities, with a particular focus on the syndemic of HIV and tuberculosis.[2] A recent article in the *New Yorker* entitled "The Hot Spotters" described a similar community-focused program that showed the cost-effectiveness of such an approach in the long run (Gawande 2011).

The final question attends to the risk that biomedicine may actually worsen syndemic interactions. This problem is compounded within the current U.S. political context, as Congress continues to shave off layer upon layer of the U.S. safety net and specifically reduces critical mental health and social services.[3] I posit that the reduction of these critical services that provide opportunities to address the social and psychological factors interacting syndemically with diabetes among the poor may facilitate increasing rates of diabetes onset, morbidity, and mortality among already marginalized populations.

The need to address the social dimension of syndemics within the clinical setting is no more evident than in the ways in which women understood diabetes and its increasing social significance in their lives. For instance, when Teresa deemed diabetes to be "part of our life," she pointed to the significance that diabetes had among her friends and family in addition to the commonness with which the disease was regarded. This reference echoes Domenga's narrative as well, where she emphasized the importance of "going on with life again." This trope illustrates that although some women found the initial diabetes diagnosis to be stressful, many eventually accepted, or simply ignored, their disease as time went on. In a sense, diabetes became one of the many stresses women packed into their "luggages." This shows how the clustering of diabetes within a population may facilitate a sort of normalization of the disease as just one form of stress among others. In this way, diabetes becomes something that is not only a physical pain, but also a social disturbance that interacts intrinsically with other social and psychological dimensions of life.

Implications for Syndemics

Understanding the interplay of structural and symbolic *V*iolence, feelings of social *I*solation, *D*epression, *D*iabetes, and *A*buse provides a general framework that extends well beyond the experience of Mexican immigrant women in Chicago and elucidates sources of suffering that function as major contributors to diabetes and its clustering with depression among the poor in the Americas. Yet, the translatability of the VIDDA Syndemic presents challenges that must not be underestimated. When translating the general VIDDA Syndemic framework to a new population, one must consider how unique historical and social factors shape the syndemic cofactors. For example, there is evidence to suggest that within the Chicago context the VIDDA Syndemic afflicts low-income Puerto Rican and African American women similarly, as these two populations have rates of diabetes and depression comparable to those of people of Mexican descent. However, subtle particularities within each population define each cofactor. For example, a major variation of the VIDDA Syndemic for Puerto Ricans lies in the fact that documentation issues do not affect immigration stress, which is a major factor for Mexican immigrants. This does not mean that Puerto Ricans might not experience feelings of social isolation as a result of relocating to Chicago, but the stress of "illegality" is not a part of their lives. In addition, the experiences of African American women in Chicago may vary due to the legacy of racism and marginalization of this group within the city, which is distinct from—though sometimes interrelated with—that of Mexican immigrants.

The VIDDA Syndemic framework also provides some insight into future projections of diabetes among the poor worldwide. For example, as I described in the introduction, the political-economic and social forces that contribute to the onset and complications of diabetes in high-income countries differ from those in low- and middle-income countries, where diabetes clusters among those who are wealthier rather than among the poor (World Health Organization 2009). As the diabetes burden shifts within poorer countries, the double burden of disease, where the onset of chronic diseases like diabetes occur in tandem with the scourge of infectious diseases like malaria, will have an impact on the syndemics of distress and diabetes (see Baer and Singer 2008). Moreover, syndemic interactions occurring at the biological level between, for example, diabetes and tuberculosis (Kant 2003; Ponce de Leon et al. 2004; Alisjahbana et al. 2006; Perez, Brown, and Restrepo 2006) will become crippling for those populations where these diseases cluster. Identifying these potential risks now and planning to mitigate their estimated effects on poor populations, and poor countries at large, is critical.

Finally, taking the VIDDA Syndemic seriously is essential for addressing issues like health inequity and the biology of poverty in the United States. Throughout this book I have described layer-upon-layer of VIDDA Syndemic interactions with the intention not only to demonstrate the synergistic interface of social suffering with depression and diabetes, but also to bring to light the critical need for comprehensive health care for the poor. In a country in which great wealth often overshadows and perpetuates great inequalities, the lack of attention to comprehensive, integrated health care for the poor is unacceptable. We may be hopeful that new national plans for comprehensive health insurance coverage, which include some of the very poor (though not the undocumented), may improve the devastating outcomes revealed in these pages. And, indeed, it can be a start. However, until biomedicine recognizes the necessity to tend to the mind, the emotions, and to the fuller experience of social suffering to effectively tend to the body, the great health disparities between those who have much and those who have much less will continue to be one of the United States' greatest hypocrisies.

NOTES

Introduction

1. All names used are pseudonyms.
2. Briefly, neoliberalism describes a market-driven approach to economic and social policy based on neoclassical economic theories, which became hegemonic during the Reagan-Thatcher era. According to neoliberal ideology, the invisible hand of the market will provide for the efficiency of private enterprise, defined by liberalized trade with relatively unregulated markets; therefore, maximizing the role of the private sector will enhance the political and economic priorities of the state. Neoliberal economic policies have contributed to the loss of skilled jobs in the heavy industry (such as steel), and to their replacement with more flexible, unskilled, and often immigrant labor in smaller factories and in the service sector (see Harvey 2005). The loss of these jobs and the transformation of power associated with wage-earning potential among low-income workers are major outcomes of neoliberalism that affect the lives and livelihoods of the women in this study. Such deterioration of power within the labor sector parallels an escalation of violence within the domestic sphere (Bourgois 2009), encapsulating the loss of social protection, fear of deportation among immigrants, and increase of poverty and marginalization of the poor in Chicago.
3. The data used for this correlation and Figure 1 were developed using data from the Centers for Disease Control and Prevention and a paper from *The Monthly Labor Review* published by the U.S. Bureau of Labor Statistics. Date (Gini, Db%): 1981 (0.369, 2.51); 1986 (0.392, 2.78); 1990 (0.396, 2.52); 1994 (0.426, 2.98); 1999 (0.428, 4.00); 2001 (0.435, 4.75). During the twenty years between 1981 and 2001 there was a 17.9 percent change in family income inequality and 43 percent change in diabetes prevalence (5.65 million to 13.11 million people). I found a strong and significant correlation ($ß = 0.81$; $p < 0.05$) between these data.
4. American Indians have the highest prevalence of type 2 diabetes in the United States at around 15 percent. These high rates cluster on U.S. reservations and are rarely found in the urban neighborhoods in Chicago where this study takes place.
5. Dr. Merrill Singer maintains an updated list of all scholarship on syndemics on Wikipedia under "Syndemic," heading "Further Reading." Refer there for an up-to-date list of references on syndemics.

Chapter 1

1. Dr. Elizabeth Jacobs has conducted extensive research on the critical role of interpreters for non-English speaking patients. She has documented that interpreter services are not only more cost-effective, but they also significantly improve quality of care and health outcomes (see Jacobs, Sadowsky, and Rathouz 2007).

2. This information was extremely difficult to retrieve. Sam del Pozo, who worked with Dr. Elizabeth Jacobs when I conducted my research, searched for this information for about a month in 2011. These data are based on that research and the information provided to him. It is not hard data collected by the County or information easily accessible to the public.

3. These data are based on personal communications with Dr. Elizabeth Jacobs in 2008.

4. Study participants were compensated $40 for their time; the shortest interview was two hours, the longest interview was six hours, and the average time was around three hours.

5. Diabetes duration was calculated by subtracting the individual's age when she was diagnosed with diabetes from her current age.

6. Diabetes severity was measured by asking each woman if she had suffered from one of six diabetes symptoms in the past four weeks—pins and needles in both feet, hypoglycemia (including sweating, weakness, anxiety, trembling, hunger, or headache), limb amputation, kidney problems, retinopathy, and neuropathy. This variable was generated as a number from one to six.

7. Diabetes distress was measured by asking five key questions from the Diabetes Distress Scale and asking participants to give a rating of one (not at all) to six (all the time) (Polonsky et al. 2005). Questions from the Diabetes Distress Scale included in this study are: 1) Feeling that diabetes is taking up too much of my mental and physical energy; 9) Feeling angry, scared, and/or depressed when I think about living with diabetes; 17) Feeling that diabetes controls my life; 21) Feeling that I will end up with serious long-term complications, no matter what I do; and 25) Feeling overwhelmed by the demands of living with diabetes. This variable was entered into regression analyses as the mean of the responses to these five questions.

8. At the beginning of the interview study participants responded to a general Health Beliefs Questionnaire (Schwab, Meyer, and Merrell 1994) and the Self-Care Inventory—Revised version (SCI-R), which was utilized to evaluate dietary patterns, activity patterns, and medication adherence (Morisky, Green, and Levine 1986; Toobert, Hampson, and Glasgow 2000).

9. I measured depression by administering the Center for Epidemiological Studies Depression Scale (CES-D). The CES-D is a widely used twenty-item questionnaire in English designed to assess the major symptoms of depression, and has been validated in Spanish (Radloff 1977; Soler et al. 1997). The CES-D's targeted symptoms include depressed mood, changes in appetite and sleep, low energy, feelings of hopelessness, low self-esteem, and loneliness. Respondents were asked to consider the presence and duration of each item/symptom over the past week and to rate each along a 4-point scale from 0 (rarely or never) to 3 (most or all of the time). Possible scores range from 0 to 60. A score of ≥ 16 is the most common cutoff point, indicating a "likely depression," and a score of ≥ 24 is often used as a more rigorous measure of "likely depression"; scores lower than these cutoff points were considered "no depression."

10. I measured Post-Traumatic Stress Disorder by administering the PTSD-Checklist Civilian Version (PCL-C). The PCL-C is a widely used seventeen-item

questionnaire designed to assess key symptoms of PTSD in the general population, in both English and Spanish (Campbell et al. 1999; Miles, Marshall, and Schell 2008). A freely available instrument adapted from the PCL-M (military), the questionnaire includes as key symptoms of PTSD: having repeated, disturbing memories and dreams; feeling as though the stressful event were happening again; feeling upset and having physical reactions to events that remind of the past; having trouble sleeping and remembering events; feeling distant from family and friends; and feeling jumpy or hyper-vigilant. These seventeen symptoms were taken directly from the DSM criteria. Respondents were asked to consider the presence and duration of each symptom over the past month and to rate each along a 5-point scale from 1 (not at all) to 5 (extremely). Possible scores ranged from 17 to 85. A score of ≥ 30 is the recommended cutoff point in a civilian primary care setting, indicating a "PTSD diagnosis," opposed to the screening cutoff point of 25 (Walker et al. 2002; Sherman et al. 2005). Scores lower than 30 were considered "no or few symptoms."

11. Anthropometrics, including height and weight, were collected at the end of the interview, and the body mass index was generated based on these measurements. Waist circumference was also measured using a standard seamstress tape measure. Systolic and diastolic blood pressures were evaluated using a standard blood pressure monitor used in medical settings.

12. Hemoglobin (Hb) A1c was derived from the dried blood spots through analysis conducted by Flexsite Diagnostics. Hemoglobin A1c, also known as glycosylated hemoglobin, has become a standard measurement for glycemic control in both clinic- and population-based studies. Glycosylated hemoglobin is formed through non-enzymatic binding of circulating glucose to hemoglobin (glycation) and is measured as the ratio of glycosylated to nonglycosylated hemoglobin (Peterson et al. 1998; Gomero et al. 2008). The rationale for this biological marker of glycemic control is based on the fairly stable level of glycosylated hemoglobin over the entire 90–120 day life span of the red blood cell (Kirkpatrick 2000). Therefore, in contrast to simply measuring glucose levels at the time of the blood spot or serum measurement, HbA1c may be interpreted as an average of the blood glucose present over the past three to four months (Peterson et al. 1998; McCarter, Hempe, and Chalew 2006).

13. Michoacán is one of thirty-one states in Mexico, located in western Mexico and bordered by Colima and Jalisco to the northwest, Guanajuato and Querétaro to the north, México to the east, Guerrero to the southeast, and the Pacific Ocean to the southwest. A large number of immigrants from Michoacán settle in Chicago.

14. A small number were English-only speakers.

15. The cutoff for poor diabetes control that I use here is based on the American Diabetic Association cutoff for hemoglobin A1c of 6.5%. In the biomedical literature, a cutoff of 8.0% is commonly used; according to this cutoff, 63% (n = 76) of the sample had poorly controlled diabetes.

Chapter 2

1. Refer to endnotes from chapter 1 (numbers 9 and 10) for a detailed description of The Center for Epidemiological Studies Depression Scale (CES-D) and PTSD-Checklist Civilian Version (PCL-C).

2. Domenga's English was somewhat conversational, but she had difficulty understanding English and communicated primarily in Spanish.

Chapter 3

1. Narrative themes were recorded into a database as dichotomous variables (0, 1). The key subthemes were defined as follows: 1) *Interpersonal abuse* reflected any behavior designated to control and/or subjugate another human being through the use of language, emotion (such as neglect), and physical or sexual violence. "Any abuse" was coded as an inclusive measure of any mention of emotional, verbal, physical, or sexual abuse. "Physical abuse" was coded as any mention of childhood physical abuse or spousal abuse. In most cases women were the victims, and in some cases they were also the perpetrators. "Sexual abuse" was coded as any mention of sexual abuse; most of these responses were childhood sexual abuse; 2) *Loss of a family member* denotes the loss of a child, of a parent or partner, and the recent loss of a relative; 3) *Feelings of social isolation and loneliness* was coded when women explicitly mentioned feeling lonely a great deal of the time; 4) *Health stress* represents women's mention of physical stress in their lives; this included the cross-cutting impact of psychological distress, physical health, diabetes-related stress, and other physical manifestations of stress such of chronic pain or cancer; 5) *Family stress* was recorded when the study participants described a disorder within the family as a stressor; the majority of these cases involved disapproval of a family member's behavior, and they were often associated with exposure to drugs, alcohol, and gangs in the neighborhood; 6) *Neighborhood violence* was considered a category of its own, registered when gang- and drug-related violence was mentioned as the cause of severe physical and/or emotional trauma or stress either in present or in the past; 7) *Immigration stress* was coded when the study participant mentioned stress associated with immigration to Chicago (border crossing, deportation) or with being an immigrant (racism); 8) *Financial stress* was only coded as such when the study participant specifically mentioned it as a strain in her life; 9) *Workplace stress* was coded when an interlocutor mentioned distress associated with discrimination and/or mistreatment in the workplace.

   First, I conducted simple correlations among narrative themes (Table 3.1) and between narrative themes and markers of immigration stress (Table 3.2). These correlations provided important insights into the interthematic interactions at play, as many women reported more than one narrative theme.

2. Diabetes stress alone was captured by two other measures: the Diabetes Distress Scale (social, psychological) and hemoglobin A1c (biological).

3. The age of immigration is measured by the average years lived in the United States (27 years, SD +/– 15).

4. The Acculturation Rating Scale for Mexican Americans (ARSMA)-II is a culturally specific scale developed to assess a number of factors including a) language use and preference; b) ethnic identity; c) cultural heritage and ethnic behaviors; and d) ethnic interaction (Cueller, Arnold, and Maldonado 1995). This scale addresses preferences (such as "I enjoy listening to Spanish language music") with a 1-5 Likert scale from "not at all" to "very much."

Chapter 4

1. An earlier version of Mari's story was presented in Mendenhall et al. (2010).

2. Mari's PCL-C score was 41, her CES-D score was 25, her BMI was 59, and HbA1c was 13.

3. Extrapolated further, 16 percent (13 of 79) of the women who immigrated from Mexico relayed immigration stories that intersected with physical and/or sexual violence.

4. A more extensive discussion of the history of U.S.-Mexican immigration can be found in De Genova's *Working the Boundaries*, especially chapter 2, entitled "The 'Native's Point of View.'"

5. Yolanda spoke proudly about her siblings' success. She stated that they did not endure abuse as children and left home as soon as they could, returning rarely. Her siblings both live outside of the Midwest, and neither has mental or physical health problems. Yolanda said proudly that her sister works as a nurse at a prestigious University Hospital on the East Coast.

6. Yolanda weighed 124 pounds, her body mass index was 22, and her diabetes control was 5.3 (HbA1c); she had severe PTSD (PCL-C: 52) and severe depression (CES-D: 41).

Chapter 5

1. There are three key physiological facts behind the developmental origins hypothesis. First, individuals who are born small have a reduced muscle mass, which lowers their energetic requirements. This fact is important because the amount of muscle that an individual has largely determines the amount of energy used during activity or while at rest. Second, low birthweight babies have greater energetic storage per unit of body mass, which results in greater fat mass. Third, abdominal fat cells are more sensitive to hormonal signals that cause the release of fats into the bloodstream among individuals who are born small, resulting in easier access to fat stores during caloric shortfalls (see Kuzawa 2008; Trevathan, Smith, and McKenna 2008).

2. For more information about the biology of stress and poverty, refer to Robert Sapolsky's *Why Zebras Don't Get Ulcers* (2004). Chapters 3, 4, 8–14, and 17 are particularly relevant for the discussion here.

3. Clinical samples generally have higher rates of psychological distress when compared to the general population. Therefore, the data regarding PTSD prevalence should be compared to general population estimates with the recognition that rates will be higher regardless. The data about veteran populations are estimated based on clinical samples.

4. No adjustment is made for multiple comparisons, as here I present the effects, confidence intervals, and p-values.

5. In Model 1 I examine the relationship of abuse with depression; in Model 2 I examine the relationship while adjusting for feeling socially detached; in Models 3 and 4 I examine the relationship between abuse and depression while adjusting for health stress and diabetes distress, respectively; in the final model I adjust for all stressors. All models were adjusted for age, income, education, language, acculturation, and BMI. Although I anticipated presenting disaggregated data for physical abuse and sexual abuse, because the results for sexual and physical abuse were so similar to "any abuse," only the data for the inclusive "any abuse" category are presented. These methods and logistic regression analyses of these data are published in *Culture, Medicine, and Psychiatry* (Mendenhall and Jacobs 2012).

6. The first three processes are explained in depth in Musselman et al. (2003).

7. Refer to Robert Sapolsky (2004) for a more extensive and engaging discussion.
8. Adam Koon was integral to the design and organization of this model. The model was influenced in part by Rosa Gonzalez-Guarda and colleagues' syndemic model (Gonzalez-Guarda, Florom-Smith, and Thomas 2011).

Conclusion

1. Teresa was a Spanish-only speaker and met with one of the two Spanish-speaking psychiatrists available.
2. Merrill Singer's *An Introduction to Syndemics* provides a more extensive discussion under the subheading: "Biomedicine and the Social Origins of Syndemics" (2009a, 208).
3. During the period of time that I was associated with the County hospital, hundreds of jobs were lost, and at one point almost half of the outlying county clinics were closed due to financial problems (beginning in 2006). The interim director of the hospital stated that hiring an additional cardiologist and gynecological oncologist would have enabled them to meet the needs of the community without need for these established clinics nestled in the center of needy communities. Similarly, there was discussion of shutting down prevention programs that focused on screening for breast and cervical cancers. This shows that safety-net systems struggling to finance themselves tend to focus on curative services as opposed to preventative ones, in spite of the well-established evidence that curative services (or "band-aid solutions") are not an effective way to deal with chronic disease. Unfortunately, these decisions are made based on financial sense as opposed to the critical social, psychological, and physical needs of the poor.

REFERENCES

Abraido-Lanza, A., M. Chao, and K. R. Flórez. 2005. Do healthy behaviors decline with greater acculturation? Implications for the Latino mortality paradox. *Social Science & Medicine* 61(6): 1243–55.

Alisjahbana, B., R. van Crevel, E. Sahiratmadja, M. den Heijer, and A. Maya. 2006. Diabetes mellitus is strongly associated with tuberculosis in Indonesia. *International Journal of Tuberculosis and Lung Disease* 10: 696–700.

Amaro, H., and A. de laTorre. 2002. Public health needs and scientific opportunities in research on Latinas. *American Journal of Public Health* 92(4): 525–29.

Anderson, R. J., K. E. Freedland, R. E. Clouse, and P. J. Lustman. 2001. The prevalence of comorbid depression in adults with diabetes. *Diabetes Care* 24: 1069–78.

Anzaldúa, G. 1987. *Borderlands/La Frontera*. San Francisco: Aunt Lute Books.

Arcia, E., M. Skinner, D. Bailey, and V. Correa. 2001. Models of acculturation and health behaviors among Latino immigrants to the U.S. *Social Science & Medicine* 53(1): 41–53.

Arredondo, G. F. 2008. *Mexican Chicago: Race, Identity, and Nation, 1916–39*. Chicago: University of Illinois Press.

Arredondo, G. F., and D. Vaillant. 2004. Mexicans. *The Encyclopedia of Chicago*. Chicago: The Newberry Library.

Arroyo, C., F. B. Hu, L. M. Ryan, I. Kawachi, G. A. Colditz, F. E. Speizer, and J. Manson. 2004. Depressive symptoms and risk of type 2 diabetes in women. *Diabetes Care* 27: 129–33.

Atkinson, P. 1990. *The Ethnographic Imagination: Textual Constructs of Reality*. New York: Routledge.

Austin, J. L. 1961. *How To Do Things with Words: The William James Lectures Delivered at Harvard University in 1955*. Edited by J. O. Urmson. Oxford: Clarendon.

Baer, H. A., and M. Singer. 2008. *Global Warming and the Political Ecology of Health: Emerging Crises and Systemic Solutions*. Walnut Creek, CA: Left Coast Press.

Baker, C., F. Norris, D. M. Diaz, J. L. Perilla, A. D. Murphy, and E. G. Hill. 2005. Violence and PTSD in Mexico: Gender and regional differences. *Social Psychiatry and Psychiatric Epidemiology* 40(7): 519–28.

Baker, C., F. H. Norris, E. C. Jones, and A. D. Murphy. 2009. Childhood trauma and adulthood physical health in Mexico. *Journal of Behavioral Medicine* 32: 255–69.

Baker, J., M. Hurtado, O. Pearson, and T. Jones. 2008. Evolutionary medicine and obesity: Developmental adaptive responses in human body composition. In *Evolutionary Medicine and Health*, eds. W. R. Trevathan, E. O. Smith, and J. J. McKenna, 314–24. Oxford: Oxford University Press.

Barker, D. J., P. D. Winter, C. Osmond, B. Margetts, and S. J. Simmonds. 1989. Weight in infancy and death from ischaemic heart disease. *Lancet* 2: 577–80.

Barker, D. J., A. R. Bull, C. Osmond, and S. J. Simmonds. 1990. Fetal and placental size and risk of hypertension in adult life. *BMJ* 301: 259–62.

Barker, D. J. 1995. Fetal origins of coronary heart disease. *BMJ* 311: 171–74.

Barker, D. J. 1999. Fetal origins of type 2 diabetes mellitus. *Annual Review of Internal Medicine* 130: 322–24.

Bauman, R. 1986. *Story, Performance, and Event*. Cambridge: Cambridge University Press.

Beaulac, J., E. Kristjansson, and S. Cummins. 2009. A systematic review of food deserts, 1966–2007. *Preventing Chronic Diseases* 6(3): A105–15.

Becker, G. 1997. *Disrupted Lives: How People Create Meaning in a Chaotic World*. Berkeley: University of California Press.

BeLue, R., T. A. Okoror, J. Iwelunmor, K. D. Taylor, A. N. Degboe, C. Agyemang, and G. Ogedegbe. 2009. An overview of cardiovascular risk factor burden in sub-Saharan African countries: A socio-cultural perspective. *Global Health* 22(5): 10–22.

Benson, M. L., J. Wooldredge, A. B. Thistlethwaite, and G. L. Fox. 2004. The correlation between race and domestic violence is confounded with community context. *Social Problems* 51(3): 326–42.

Berkman, L. F., and S. L. Syme. 1979. Social networks, host resistance, and mortality: A nine-year follow-up study of Alameda County residents. *American Journal of Epidemiology* 109(2): 186–204.

Berkman, L. F., T. Glass, I. Brissettec, and T. E. Seeman. 2000. From social integration to health: Durkheim in the new millennium. *Social Science & Medicine* 51: 843–57.

Bermudez, O., L. Falcon, and K. L. Tucker. 2000. Intake and food sources of macronutrients among older Hispanic adults: Association with ethnicity, acculturation, and length of residence in the United States. *Journal of the American Dietetic Association* 100(6): 665–73.

Bernard, H. R. 1988. *Research Methods in Cultural Anthropology*. Newbury Park, CA: Sage.

Berry, J. 1970. Marginality, stress and ethnic identification in an acculturated Aboriginal community. *Journal of Cross-Cultural Psychology* 1: 239–52.

Berry, J. 1990. Psychology of acculturation. In *Nebraska Symposium on Motivation, Vol. 37: Cross-cultural Perspectives*, ed. J. J. Berman, 201–34. Lincoln: University of Nebraska Press.

Berry, J. 1997. Immigration, acculturation, and adaptation. *Applied Psychology: An International Review* 46(1): 5–68.

Berry, J. 1998. Acculturation and health: Theory and research. In *Cultural Clinical Psychology: Theory, Research, and Practice*, eds. S. S. Kazarian and D. R. Evans, 39–57. New York: Oxford University Press.

Berry, J. 2003. Conceptual approaches to acculturation. In *Acculturation: Advances in Theory, Measurement, and Applied Research*, eds. K. Chun, P. Balls Organista, and G. Marin, 17–37. Washington, DC: American Psychological Association.

Birch, L. 1987. The acquisition of food acceptance patterns in children. In *Eating Habits: Food, Physiology, and Learned Behaviour*, eds. R. A. Boakes, D. A. Popplewell, and M. J. Burton, 107–30. Chichester, UK: John Wiley & Sons.

Bishaw, A., and J. Iceland. 2003. *Poverty: 1999. Census 2000 Brief.* Washington, DC: United States Census Bureau. http://www.census.gov/prod/2003pubs/c2kbr-19.pdf.

Black, P. 2003. The inflammatory response is an integral part of the stress response: Implications for atherosclerosis, insulin resistance, type II diabetes and metabolic syndrome X. *Brain Behavior and Immunity* 17: 350–64.

Black, S. A., K. S. Markides, and L. A. Ray. 2003. Depression predicts increased incidence of adverse health outcomes in older Mexican Americans with type 2 diabetes. *Diabetes Care* 26: 2822–28.

Borrell, L., N. Crawford, F. J. Dallo, and M. C. Baquero. 2009. Self-reported diabetes in Hispanic subgroup, non-Hispanic black, and non-Hispanic white populations: National Health Interview Survey, 1997–2005. *Public Health Reports* 124(5): 702–10.

Bourdieu, P. 1989. Social space and symbolic power. *Sociological Theory* 7(1): 18–26.

Bourdieu, P. 2001. *Masculine Domination.* Palo Alto, CA: Stanford University Press.

Bourdieu, P., and L. Wacquant. 2004. Symbolic violence. In *Violence in War and Peace: An Anthology*, eds. N. Scheper-Hughes and P. Bourgois, 272–74. Malden, MA: Blackwell Publishing.

Bourgois, P. 1998. The moral economies of homeless heroin addicts: Confronting ethnography, HIV risk, and everyday violence in San Francisco shooting encampments. *Substance Use and Misuse* 33(11): 2323–51.

Bourgois, P. 2001. The power of violence in war and peace: Post-cold war lessons from El Salvador. *Ethnography* 2(1): 5–37.

Bourgois, P. 2009. Recognizing invisible violence. In *Global Health in Times of Violence*, eds. B. Rylko-Bauer, L. Whiteford, and P. Farmer, 17–40. Santa Fe, NM: School for Advanced Research Press.

Bourgois, P., B. Prince, and A. Moss. 2004. The everyday violence of hepatitis C among young women who inject drugs in San Francisco. *Human Organization* 63(3): 253–64.

Boyce, T., and E. Chesterman. 1990. Life events, social support, and cardiovascular reactivity in adolescence. *Developmental and Behavioral Pediatrics* 11(3): 105–11.

Breslau, N., G. Davis, P. Andreski, E. L. Peterson, and L. R. Schultz. 1997. Sex differences in posttraumatic stress disorder. *Archives of General Psychiatry* 54: 1044–48.

Briere, J., and D. M. Elliot. 2003. Prevalence and psychological sequelae of self-reported childhood physical and sexual abuse in a general population sample of men and women. *Child Abuse & Neglect* 27(10): 1205–22.

Bromet, E., A. Sonnega, and R. C. Kessler. 1998. Risk factors for DSM-III-R posttraumatic stress disorder: Findings from the National Comorbidity Survey. *American Journal of Epidemiology* 147: 353–61.

Bruner, J. 1986. *Actual Minds, Possible Worlds*. Cambridge: Harvard University Press.

Campbell, K., D. Rohlman, D. Storzbach, L. M. Binder, W. K. Anger, C. A. Kovera, K. L. Davis, and S. J. Grossman. 1999. Test-retest reliability of psychological and neurobehavioral tests self-administered by computer. *Assessment* 6(1): 21–32.

Capps, L., and E. Ochs. 1995. *Constructing Panic: A Discourse on Agoraphobia*. Cambridge: Harvard University Press.

Carnethon, M., L. Kinder, J. M. Fair, R. S. Stafford, and S. P. Fortmann. 2003. Symptoms of depression as risk factor for incident diabetes: Findings from the national health and nutrition examination of epidemiologic follow-up study, 1971–1992. *American Journal of Epidemiology* 158: 416–23.

Castañeda, H. 2010. Im/migration and health: Conceptual, methodological, and theoretical propositions for applied anthropology. *NAPA Bulletin* 34: 6–27.

Centers for Disease Control and Prevention (CDC). 2010. Age-Adjusted Percentage of Civilian, Noninstitutionalized Population with Diagnosed Diabetes, Hispanics, United States, 1997–2008. Division of Health Interview Statistics, National Health Interview Survey.

Chock, P. P. 1996. No new women: Gender, "alien," and "citizen" in the congressional debate on immigration. *PoLAR: Political and Legal Anthropology Review* 19(1): 1–9.

Chrousos, G. P., and P. W. Gold. 1992. The concepts of stress and stress system disorders: Overview of physical and behavioral homeostasis. *Journal of the American Medical Association* 267(9): 1244–52.

Clark, L., D. Vincent, L. Zimmer, and J. Sanchez. 2009. Cultural values and political economic contexts of diabetes among low-income Mexican Americans. *Journal of Transcultural Nursing* 20(4): 382–94.

Cohen, S., and G. M. Williamson. 1988. Stress and infectious disease in humans. *Psychological Bulletin* 109: 5–24.

Cordain, L. 1999. Cereal grains: Humanity's double-edged sword. *World Review of Nutrition and Dietetics* 84: 19–73.

Cowie, C. C., K. F. Rust, D. D. Byrd-Holt, E. W. Gregg, E. S. Ford, L. S. Geiss, K. E. Bainbridge, and J. E. Fradkin. 2010. Prevalence of diabetes and high risk for diabetes using A1C criteria in the U.S. population in 1988–2006. *Diabetes Care* 33: 562–68.

Cristancho, S., M. Garces, K. E. Peters, and B. C. Mueller. 2008. Listening to rural Hispanic immigrants in the Midwest: Community-based participatory assessment of major barriers to health care access and use. *Qualitative Health Research* 18(5): 633–46.

Cueller, I., B. Arnold, and R. Maldonado. 1995. Acculturation rating scale for Mexican Americans II. *Hispanic Journal of Behavioral Sciences* 17(3): 275–304.

Dalal, S., J. J. Beunza, J. Volmink, C. Adebamowo, F. Bajunirwe, M. Nielekela, D. Mozaffarian, W. Fawzi, W. Willett, H. O. Adami, and M. D. Holmes. 2011. Non-communicable diseases in sub-Saharan Africa: What we know now. *International Journal of Epidemiology* 40(4): 885–901.

Dandona, P., A. Aljada, and A. Bandyopadhyay. 2004. Inflammation: The link between insulin resistance, obesity and diabetes. *Trends in Immunology* 25(1): 4–7.

De Genova, N. 2005. *Working the Boundaries: Race, Space, and "Illegality" in Mexican Chicago.* Durham, NC: Duke University Press.

De Genova, N., and A. Y. Ramos-Zayas. 2003. *Latino Crossings: Mexicans, Puerto Ricans, and the Politics of Race and Citizenship.* New York: Routledge.

De Genova, N., and N. M. Peutz. 2010. *The Deportation Regime: Sovereignty, Space, and the Freedom of Movement.* Durham, NC: Duke University Press.

de Groot, M., R. J. Anderson, K. E. Freedland, R. E. Clouse, and P. J. Lustman. 2001. Association of depression and diabetes complications: A meta-analysis. *Psychosomatic Medicine* 63: 619–30.

de Groot, M., B. Pinkerman, J. Wagner, and E. Hockman. 2006. Depression treatment and satisfaction in a multicultural sample of type 1 and type 2 diabetic patients. *Diabetes Care* 29: 549–53.

de la Torre, A., R. Frus, H. R. Hunter, and L. Garcia. 1996. The health insurance status of U.S. Latino women: A profile from the 1982–1984 Hispanic HANES. *American Journal of Public Health* 86: 534–37.

Dixon, L., J. Sundquist, and M. A. Winkleby. 2000. Differences in energy, nutrient, and food intakes in a U.S. sample of Mexican-American women and men: Findings from the Third National Health and Nutrition Examination Survey, 1988–1994. *American Journal of Epidemiology* 152(6): 548–57.

Dohrenwend, B. S., B. P. Dohrenwend, M. Dodson, and P. E. Shrout. 1984. Symptoms, hassles, social supports, and life events: Problem of confounded measures. *Journal of Abnormal Psychology* 93(2): 222–30.

Dohrenwend, B., J. B. Turner, N. A. Turse, B. G. Adams, K. C. Koenen, and R. Marshall. 2006. The psychological risks of Vietnam for U.S. veterans: A revisit with new data and methods. *Science* 313: 979.

Dong, M., R. F. Anda, V. J. Felitti, S. R. Dube, D. F. Williamson, T. J. Thompson, C. M. Loos, and W. H. Giles. 2004. The interrelatedness of multiple forms of childhood abuse, neglect, and household dysfunction. *Child Abuse and Neglect* 28(7): 771–84.

Dressler, W. 1993. Health in the African American community: Accounting for health inequalities. *Medical Anthropology Quarterly* 73: 25–34.

Eaton, S. B., M. Shostak, and M. Konner. 1988. *The Paleolithic Prescription.* New York: Harper & Row.

Eaton, S. B., S. B. I. Eaton, and L. Cordain. 2002. Evolution, diet, and health. In *Human Diet: Its Origin and Evolution*, eds. P. S. Ungar and M. F. Teaford, 7–17. Westport, CT: Bergin & Garvey.

Egede, L., and C. Ellis. 2010. Diabetes and depression: Global perspectives. *Diabetes Research and Clinical Practice* 87: 302–12.

Epel, E. S., B. McEwen, T. Seeman, K. Matthews, G. Castellazzo, K. D. Brownell, J. Bell, and J. R. Ickovics. 2000. Stress and body shape: Stress-induced cortisol secretion is consistently greater among women with central fat. *Psychosomatic Medicine* 62: 623–32.

Epel, E. S., R. Lapidus, B. McEwen, and K. Brownell. 2001. Stress may add bite to appetite in women: A laboratory study of stress-induced cortisol and eating behavior. *Psychoneuroendocrinology* 26: 37–49.

Eschbach, K., G. Ostir, K. V. Patel, K. S. Markides, and J. S. Goodwin. 2004. Neighborhood context and mortality among older Mexican Americans: Is there a barrio advantage? *American Journal of Public Health* 94(10): 1807–12.

Escobar, J. I., C. Hoyos Nervi, and M. A. Gara. 2000. Immigration and mental health: Mexican Americans in the United States. *Harvard Review of Psychiatry* 8: 64–72.

Everson-Rose, S., J. Torrens, P. M. Meyer, H. M. Kravitz, L. H. Powell, J. T. Bromberger, D. Pandey, and K. A. Matthews. 2004. Depressive symptoms, insulin resistance, and risk of diabetes in women at midlife. *Diabetes Care* 27: 2856–62.

Ewald, P. 2008. An evolutionary perspective on the causes of chronic diseases: Atherosclerosis as an illustration. In *Evolutionary Medicine and Health*, eds. W. R. Trevathan, E. O. Smith, and J. J. McKenna, 350–67. Oxford: Oxford University Press.

Farley, T., A. Galves, M. Dickinson, and M. J. Diaz Perez. 2005. Stress, coping, and health: A comparison of Mexican immigrants, Mexican-Americans, and non-Hispanic whites. *Journal of Immigrant Health* 7(3): 213–20.

Farmer, P. 1997. On suffering and structural violence: A view from below. In *Social Suffering*, eds. A. Kleinman, V. Das, and M. M. Lock, 261–83. Berkeley: University of California Press.

Farmer, P. 1999. *Infections and Inequalities: The Modern Plagues*. Berkeley: University of California Press.

Farmer, P. 2004. An anthropology of structural violence. *Current Anthropology* 45(3): 305–25.

Farmer, P., F. Léandre, J. S. Mukherjee, M. Claude, P. Nevil, M. C. Smith-Fawzi, S. P. Koenig, A. Castro, M. C. Becerra, J. Sachs, A. Attaran, and J. Y. Kim. 2001. Community-based approaches to HIV treatment in resource-poor settings. *Lancet* 358: 404–9.

Farmer, P., B. Nizeye, S. Stulac, and S. Keshavjee. 2006. Structural violence and clinical medicine. *PLoS Medicine* 3(10): e449.

Farr, M. 2006. *Rancheros in Chicagoacán*. Austin: University of Texas Press.

Fava, M. 2000. Weight gain and antidepressants. *Journal of Clinical Psychiatry* 61(Suppl. 11): 37–41.

Felitti, V. J., R. F. Anda, D. Nordenberg, D. F. Williamson, A. M. Spitz, V. Edwards, M. P. Koss, and J. S. Marks. 1998. Relationship of childhood abuse and household dysfunction to many of the leading causes of death in adults. *American Journal of Preventive Medicine* 14: 245–58.

Finkler, K. 1994. *Women in Pain: Gender and Morbidity in Mexico*. Philadelphia: University of Philadelphia Press.

Finkler, K. 1997. Gender, domestic violence and sickness in Mexico. *Social Science & Medicine* 45(8): 1147–60.

Fisher, L., J. T. Mullan, C. Chesla, R. J. Bartz, M. M. Skaff, R. A. Kanter, C. Gilliss, and C. P. Lutz. 2000. The family and disease management in Hispanic and European-American patients with type 2 diabetes. *Diabetes Care* 23: 267–72.

Fisher, L., C. Chesla, J. Mullan, M. Skaff, and R. Kanter. 2001. Contributors to depression in Latino and European-American patients with type 2 diabetes. *Diabetes Care* 24: 1751–57.

Fisher, L., M. Skaff, J. T. Mullan, P. Arean, R. Glasgown, and U. Masharani. 2008. A longitudinal study of affective and anxiety disorders, depressive affect and diabetes distress in adults with type 2 diabetes. *Diabetic Medicine* 25(9): 1096–1101.

Ford, D., and T. Erlinger. 2004. Depression and C-reactive protein in U.S. adults: Data from the third national health and nutrition examination survey. *Archives of Internal Medicine* 164: 1010–14.

Freeman, M. 1993. *Rewriting the Self: History, Memory, Narrative*. London: Routledge.

Galtung, J. 1969. Violence, peace, and peace research. *Journal of Peace Research* 6(3): 167–91.

Garcia, J. G. A., A. Salcedo Rocha, I. Lopez, R. D. Baer, W. Dressler, and S. C. Weller. 2007. "Diabetes is my companion": Lifestyle and self-management among good and poor control Mexican diabetic patients. *Social Science & Medicine* 64: 2223–35.

Garro, L. C. 2008. Remembering what one knows and the construction of the past: A comparison of cultural knowledge of cultural consensus theory and cultural schema theory. *Ethos* 28(3): 275–319.

Garro, L. C., and C. Mattingly. 2000. Narrative as construct and construction. In *Narrative and the Cultural Construction of Illness and Healing*, eds. C. Mattingly and L. C. Garro, 1–49. Berkeley: University of California Press.

Gawande, A. 2011. The Hot Spotters: Can we lower medical costs by giving the neediest patients better care? *The New Yorker*, January 24.

Golden, S. H., B. L. H. Chang, H. B. Lee, P. J. Schreiner, A. D. Roux, A. L. Fitzpatrick, M. Szklo, and C. Lyketsos. 2007. Depression and type 2 diabetes mellitus: The multiethnic study of atherosclerosis. *Psychosomatic Medicine* 69: 529–36.

Golden, S., M. Lazo, M. Carnethon, A. G. Bertoni, P. J. Schreiner, A. V. Diez Roux, H. B. Lee, and C. Lyketsos. 2008. Examining a bidirectional association between depressive symptoms and diabetes. *Journal of the American Medical Association* 299(23): 2751–59.

Gomero, A., T. McDade, S. Williams, and S. T. Lindau. 2008. Dried blood spot measurement of glycosylated hemoglobin (HbA1c) in wave 1 of the National Social Life, Health & Aging Project. Chicago: NORC and the University of Chicago. http://biomarkers.uchicago.edu/pdfs/TR-HbA1c.pdf.

Gonzalez, H., M. Ceballos, W. Tarraf, B. T. West, M. E. Bowen, and W. A. Vega. 2009. The health of older Mexican Americans in the long run. *American Journal of Public Health* 10(99): 1879–85.

Gonzalez, H. M., W. Tarraf, K. E. Whitfield, and W. A. Vega. 2010. The epidemiology of major depression and ethnicity in the United States. *Journal of Psychiatric Research* 44(15): 1043–51.

Gonzalez-Guarda, R., A. Florom-Smith, and T. Thomas. 2011. A syndemic model of substance abuse, intimate partner violence, HIV infection, and mental health among Hispanics. *Public Health Nursing* 28(4): 366–78.

Good, B. 1977. The heart of what's the matter: The semantics of illness in Iran. *Culture, Medicine, and Psychiatry* 1: 25–58.

Good, B. 1994. *Medicine, Rationality, and Experience: An Anthropological Perspective.* Cambridge: Cambridge University Press.

Good, M.-J. D., B. Good, P. E. Brodwin, and A. Kleinman. 1992. *Pain as Human Experience: An Anthropological Perspective.* Berkeley: University of California Press.

Goode, J., and J. Maskovsky. 2001. *The New Poverty Studies.* New York: New York University Press.

Goodman, A. H., and T. L. Leatherman. 1998. *Building a New Biocultural Synthesis: Political-Economic Perspectives on Human Biology.* Ann Arbor: University of Michigan Press.

Gordon-Larsen, P., K. Harris, D. W. Ward, and B. M. Popkin. 2003. Acculturation and overweight-related behaviors among Hispanic immigrants to the U.S.: The National Longitudinal Study of Adolescent Health. *Social Science & Medicine* 57: 2023–34.

Gravlee, C., W. Dressler, and H. R. Bernard. 2005. Skin color, social classification, and blood pressure in Puerto Rico. *American Journal of Public Health* 95(12): 2191–97.

Guarnaccia, P. J. 1992. *Ataque de nervios* in Puerto Rico: Culture-bound syndrome or popular illness? *Medical Anthropology* 15: 1–14.

Guendelman, S., and B. Abrams. 1995. Dietary intake among Mexican-American women: Generational differences and a comparison with white non-Hispanic women. *American Journal of Public Health* 85(1): 20–25.

Gutmann, M. C. 1999. Ethnicity, alcohol, and acculturation. *Social Science & Medicine* 48: 173–84.

Harvey, D. 2005. *A Brief History of Neoliberalism.* Oxford: Oxford University Press.

Heilemann, M. V., F. S. Kury, and K. A. Lee. 2005. Trauma and posttraumatic stress disorder symptoms among low-income women of Mexican descent in the United States. *The Journal of Nervous and Mental Disease* 193(10): 665–72.

Herman, J. 1992. *Trauma and Recovery.* New York: Basic Books.

Himmelgreen, D. A., N. R. Daza, E. Cooper, and D. Martinez. 2007. "I don't make the soups anymore": Pre- to post-migration dietary and lifestyle changes among Latinos living in West-Central Florida. *Ecology of Food and Nutrition* 46(5–6): 427–44.

Hirsch, J. 2003a. *A Courtship After Marriage: Sexuality and Love in Mexican Transnational Families.* Berkeley: University of California Press.

Hirsch, J. 2003b. Anthropologists, migrants, and health research: Confronting cultural appropriateness. In *American Arrivals: Anthropology Engages the New Immigration*, ed. N. Foner, 229–57. Santa Fe: School of American Research Press.

Holman, E. A., R. C. Silver, and H. Waitzkin. 2000. Traumatic life events in primary care patients: A study in an ethnically diverse sample. *Archives of Family Medicine* 9(9): 802–10.

Holmes, S. 2006. An ethnographic study of the social context of migrant health in the United States. *PLoS Medicine* 3(10): e448.

Hovey, J., and C. Magana. 2000. Acculturative stress, anxiety, and depression among Mexican immigrant farmworkers in the Midwest United States. *Journal of Immigrant Health* 2(3): 119–31.

Hunt, L., S. Schneider, and B. Comer. 2004. Should "acculturation" be a variable in health research? A critical review of research on US Hispanics. *Social Science & Medicine* 59: 973–86.

Hunt, L., M. Valenzuela, and J. A. Pugh. 1998. Porque me tocó a mi? Mexican American diabetes patients' causal stories and their relationship to treatment behaviors. *Social Science & Medicine* 46(8): 959–69.

Hunt, L. M. 1998. Moral reasoning and the meaning of cancer: Causal explanations of oncologists and patients in southern Mexico. *Medical Anthropology Quarterly* 12(3): 298–318.

Hunt, L. M. 2000. Strategic suffering: Illness narratives as social empowerment among Mexican cancer patients. In *Narrative and the Construction of Illness and Healing*, eds. C. Mattingly and L. C. Garro, 88–107. Berkeley: University of California Press.

Hurwitz, T. A., C. Clark, E. Murphy, H. Klonoff, W. R. Martin, and B. Pate. 1990. Regional cerebral glucose metabolism in major depressive disorder. *Canadian Journal of Psychiatry* 35: 684–88.

International Diabetes Federation. 2009. *IDF Diabetes Atlas.* 4th edition. Brussels, Belgium: International Diabetes Federation.

Jacobs, E. A., L. S. Sadowsky, and P. J. Rathouz. 2007. The impact of an enhanced interpreter service intervention on hospital costs and patient satisfaction. *Journal of General Internal Medicine* 22(Suppl. 2): 306–11.

Jezewski, M., and J. Poss. 2002. Mexican Americans' explanatory model of type 2 diabetes. *Western Journal of Nursing Research* 24(8): 840–58.

Johnson, D., T. Smeeding, and B. Boyle Torrey. 2005. Economic inequality through the prisms of income and consumption. *Monthly Labor Review* 128(4): 11–24.

Kant, L. 2003. Diabetes mellitus-tuberculosis: The brewing double trouble. *Indian Journal of Tuberculosis* 50(4): 83–84.

Keister, L. A., and S. Moller. 2000. Wealth inequality in the United States. *Annual Review of Sociology* 26: 63–81.

Kerr, L. A. N. 1976. The Chicago experience in Chicago: 1920–1970. PhD diss., University of Illinois at Chicago.

Kerr, L. A. N. 1977. Mexican Chicago: Chicano assimilation aborted, 1939–1954. In *Ethnic Chicago*, eds. M. G. Holli and P. d'. A. Jones, 269–98. Grand Rapids, MI: William B. Eerdmans.

Kiecolt-Glaser, J., and R. Glaser. 2002. Depression and immune function: Central pathways to morbidity and mortality. *Journal of Psychosomatic Research* 53: 873–76.

Kirby, A. P. 1991. *Narrative and the Self.* Bloomington: Indiana University Press.

Kirkpatrick, E. 2000. Glycated haemoglobin in the year 2000. *Journal of Clinical Pathology* 53(5): 335–39.

Kirmayer, L. J. 1992. The body's insistence on meaning: Metaphor as presentation and representation in illness experience. *Medical Anthropology Quarterly* 6(4): 323–46.

Kleinman, A. 1980. *Patients and Healers in the Context of Culture: An Exploration of the Borderland between Anthropology, Medicine, and Psychiatry.* Berkeley: University of California Press.

Kleinman, A. 1988. *The Illness Narratives: Suffering, Healing, and the Human Condition.* New York: Basic Books.

Kleinman, A., V. Das, and M. Lock. 1996. *Social Suffering.* Berkeley: University of California Press.

Knol, M., J. Twisk, A. T. F. Beekman, R. J. Heine, and F. Pouwer. 2006. Depression as a risk factor for the onset of type 2 diabetes mellitus: A meta-analysis. *Diabetologia* 49(5): 837–45.

Krieger, N. 1999. Embodying inequality: A review of concepts, measures, and methods for studying health consequences of discrimination. *International Journal of Health Services* 29(2): 295–352.

Krieger, N. 2005. Embodiment: A conceptual glossary for epidemiology. *Journal of Epidemiology and Community Health* 59: 350–55.

Kuzawa, C. 2008. The developmental origins of adult health: Intergenerational inertia in adaptation and disease. In *Evolutionary Medicine and Health*, eds. W. R. Trevathan, E. O. Smith, and J. J. McKenna, 325–49. Oxford: Oxford University Press.

Kuzawa, C. W., and E. Sweet. 2009. Epigenetics and the embodiment of race: Developmental origins of U.S. racial disparities in cardiovascular health. *American Journal of Human Biology* 21: 2–15.

Labov, W. 1972. *Language in the Inner City: Studies in the Black English Vernacular.* Philadelphia: University of Pennsylvania.

Lancaster, R. 1994. *Life is Hard: Machismo, Danger, and the Intimacy of Power in Nicaragua.* Berkeley: University of California Press.

Langellier, K. 2001. Personal narrative. In *Encyclopedia of Life Writing: Autobiographical and Biographical Forms*, ed. M. Jolly, 2. London: Fitzroy Dearborn.

Lara, M., C. Gamboa, M. I. Kahramanian, L. S. Morales, and D. E. Hayes Bautista. 2005. Acculturation and Latino health in the United States: A review of the literature and its sociopolitical context. *Annual Review of Public Health* 26: 367–97.

Leonard, W. R. 2001. Assessing the influence of physical activity on health and fitness. *American Journal of Human Biology* 13(2): 159–61.

Li, C., E. Ford, T. W. Strine, and A. H. Mokdad. 2008. Prevalence of depression among U.S. adults with diabetes: Findings from the 2006 Behavioral Risk Factor Surveillance System. *Diabetes Care* 31: 105–7.

Li, C., E. Ford, G. Zhao, T. W. Strine, S. Dhingra, L. Barker, J. T. Berry, and A. H. Mokdad. 2009. Association between diagnosed diabetes and serious psychological distress among U.S. adults: The Behavioral Risk Factor Surveillance System, 2007. *International Journal of Public Health* 54(Suppl. 1): 43–51.

Lieberman, L. S. 2003. Dietary, evolutionary, and modernizing influences on the prevalence of type 2 diabetes. *Annual Review of Nutrition* 23: 345–77.

Lieberman, L. S. 2006. Evolutionary and anthropological perspectives on optimal foraging in obesogenic environments. *Appetite* 47(1): 3–9.

Lieberman, L. S. 2008. Diabesity and darwinian medicine: The evolution of an epidemic. In *Evolutionary Medicine and Health*, eds. W. R. Trevathan, E. O. Smith, and J. J. McKenna, 72–95. Oxford: Oxford University Press.

Loewe, R., and J. Freeman. 2000. Interpreting diabetes mellitus: Differences between patient and provider models of disease and their implications for clinical practice. *Culture, Medicine, and Psychiatry* 24(4): 379–401.

Lown, E. A., and W. A. Vega. 2001. Prevalence and predictors of physical partner abuse among Mexican American women. *American Journal of Public Health* 91(3): 441–45.

Lustman, P. J., R. J. Anderson, K. E. Freedland, M. de Groot, R. M. Carney, and R. E. Clouse. 2000. Depression and poor glycemic control. *Diabetes Care* 23: 934–42.

Madden, S., and J. Sim. 2006. Creating meaning in fibromyalgia syndrome. *Social Science & Medicine* 63(11): 2962–73.

Marks, G., M. Garcia, and J. M. Solis. 1990. Health risk behaviors of Hispanics in the United States: Findings from HHANES, 1982–1984. *American Journal of Public Health* 80(Suppl.): 20–26.

Marmot, M., and R. G. Wilkinson. 2001. Psychosocial and material pathways in the relation between income and health: A response to Lynch et al. *British Medical Journal* 322: 1233–36.

Martinot, J. L., P. Hardy, A. Feline, J. D. Huret, B. Mazoyer, D. Attar-Levy, S. Pappata, and A. Syrota. 1990. Left prefrontal glucose metabolism in the depressed state: A confirmation. *American Journal of Psychiatry* 147: 1313–17.

Maskovsky, J., and I. Susser. 2009. Introduction: Rethinking America. In *Rethinking America: The Imperial Homeland in the 21st Century*, eds. J. Maskovsky and I. Susser, i–xii. Boulder, CO: Paradigm.

Mattingly, C. 1998. *Healing Dramas and Clinical Plots*. Cambridge: Cambridge University Press.

McAdams, D. 1996. Narrating the self in adulthood. In *Aging and Biography: Explorations in Adult Development*, ed. J. E. Birren, 131–48. New York: Springer Publishing Company.

McCarter, R., J. Hempe, and S. A. Chalew. 2006. Mean blood glucose and biological variation have greater influence on HbA1c levels than glucose instability. *Diabetes Care* 29: 352–55.

McDade, T. W. 2001. Lifestyle incongruity, social integration, and immune function in Samoan adolescents. *Social Science & Medicine* 53: 1351–62.

McDade, T. W. 2002. Status incongruity in Samoan youth: A biocultural analysis of culture change, stress, and immune function. *Medical Anthropology Quarterly* 16(2): 123–50.

McEwen, B. 2004. Protection and damage from acute and chronic stress, allostasis and allostatic load overload and relevance to the pathophysiology of psychiatric disorders. *Annals of the New York Academy of Sciences* 1032: 1–7.

McEwen, B., and T. Seeman. 1999. Protective and damaging effects of mediators of stress: Elaborating and testing the concepts of allostasis and allostatic load. In *Socioeconomic*

Status and Health in Industrial Nations: Social, Psychological and Biological Pathways, eds. N. Adler, M. Marmot, B. McEwen, and J. Stewart, 30–47. New York: New York Academy of Sciences.

McEwen, B. S. 1998. Stress, adaptation, and disease: Allostasis and allostatic load. *Annals of the New York Academy of Science* 840: 33–44.

McGarvey, S. T., J. R. Bindon, D. E. Crews, and D. E. Schendel. 1989. Modernization and adiposity: Causes and consequences. In *Human Population Biology*, eds. M. Little and J. Haas, 263–80. London: Oxford University Press.

Mendenhall, E., R. Seligman, A. Fernandez, and E. A. Jacobs. 2010. Speaking through diabetes: Rethinking the significance of lay discourses on diabetes. *Medical Anthropology Quarterly* 24(2): 220–39.

Mendenhall, E., and E. A. Jacobs. 2012. Interpersonal abuse and depression among Mexican immigrant women with type 2 diabetes. *Culture, Medicine and Psychiatry* 36(1): 136–53.

Mendenhall, E., A. Fernandez, N. Adler, and E. A. Jacobs. 2012. *Susto, coraje,* and abuse: Depression and beliefs about diabetes causality. *Culture, Medicine and Psychiatry* 36(3), pub. online April 27.

Mercado-Martinez, F. J., and I. M. Ramos-Herrera. 2002. Diabetes: The layperson's theories of causality. *Qualitative Health Research* 12(6): 792–806.

Messer, E. 1986. Some like it sweet: Estimating sweetness preferences and sucrose intakes from ethnographic and experimental data. *American Anthropologist* 88(3): 637–47.

Mezuk, B., W. Eaton, S. Albrecht, and S. H. Golden. 2008. Depression and type 2 diabetes over the lifespan: A meta-analysis. *Diabetes Care* 31: 2383–90.

Miles, J., G. Marshall, and T. L. Schell. 2008. Spanish and English versions of the PTSD Checklist-Civilian version (PCL-C): Testing for differential item functioning. *Journal of Traumatic Stress* 21(4): 368–76.

Monteiro, C., E. Moura, W. L. Conde, and B. M. Popkin. 2004. Socioeconomic status and obesity in adult populations of developing countries: A review. *Bulletin of the World Health Organization* 82: 940–46.

Montoya, M. 2011. *Making the Mexican Diabetic: Race, Science, and the Genetics of Inequality.* Berkeley: University of California Press.

Morenoff, J. D., R. J. Sampson, and S. W. Raudenbush. 2006. Neighborhood inequality, collective efficacy, and the spatial dynamics of urban violence. *Criminology* 39(3): 517–58.

Morisky, D. E., L. W. Green, and D. M. Levine. 1986. Concurrent and predictive validity of self-reported measure of medication adherence. *Medical Care* 24(1): 67–74.

Morsy, S. 1996. Political economy in medical anthropology. In *Medical Anthropology: Contemporary Theory and Method*, eds. C. F. Sargent and T. M. Johnson, 21–40. New York: Praeger.

Moscicki, E., B. Locke, D. S. Ray, and J. S. Boyd. 1989. Depressive symptoms among Mexican Americans: The Hispanic health and nutrition examination survey. *American Journal of Epidemiology* 130: 348–60.

Mullings, L. 1987. *Cities of the United States in Urban Anthropology.* New York: Columbia University Press.

Murray, C., and A. Lopez, eds. 1996. *The Global Burden of Disease: A Comprehensive Assessment of Mortality and Disability from Diseases, Injuries, and Risk Factors in 1990 and Projected to 2020.* Boston, MA: Harvard School of Public Health.

Musselman, D., E. Betan, H. Larsen, and L. S. Phillips. 2003. Relationship of depression to diabetes types 1 and 2: Epidemiology, biology, and treatment. *Biological Psychiatry* 54: 317–29.

Mustanski, B., R. Garofalo, A. Herrick, and G. Donenberg. 2007. Psychosocial health problems increase risk for HIV among urban young men who have sex with men: Preliminary evidence of a syndemic in need of attention. *Annals of Behavioral Medicine* 34: 37–45.

Narayan, K. V., J. P. Boyle, T. J. Thompson, S. W. Sorenson, and D. F. Williamson. 2003. Lifetime risk for diabetes mellitus in the United States. *Journal of the American Medical Association* 290(14): 1884–90.

Neel, J. V. 1962. Diabetes mellitus: A "thrifty genotype" rendered detrimental by "progress". *American Journal of Human Genetics* 14: 353–62.

Neel, J. V., A. B. Weder, and S. Julius. 1998. Type II diabetes, essential hypertension, and obesity as "syndromes of impaired genetic homeostasis": The "thrifty genotype" hypothesis enters the 21st century. *Perspectives in Biology and Medicine* 42: 44–74.

Neuhouser, M., B. Thompson, G. C. Coronado, and C. C. Solomon. 2004. Higher fat intake and lower fruit and vegetables intakes are associated with greater acculturation among Mexicans living in Washington State. *Journal of American Dietetic Association* 104(1): 51–57.

Nichter, M. 1981. Idioms of distress: Alternatives in the expression of psychosocial distress: A case study from South India. *Culture, Medicine and Psychiatry* 5: 379–408.

Nichter, M. 2010. Idioms of distress revisited. *Culture, Medicine and Psychiatry* 34(2): 401–16.

Nihalani, N., T. L. Schwartz, U. A. Siddiqui, and J. A. Magna. 2011. Weight gain, obesity and psychotropic prescribing. *Journal of Obesity*, pub. online January 17.

Nordstrom, C. 2004. The tomorrow of violence. In *Violence*, ed. N. L. Whitehead, 223–42. Santa Fe, NM: School of American Research Press.

Norris, S. A., C. Osmond, D. Gigante, C. W. Kuzawa, L. Ramakrishnan, N. R. Lee, M. Ramirez-Zea, L. M. Richter, A. D. Stein, N. Tandon, C.H. D. Fall, and the COHORTS Group. 2012. Size at birth, weight gain in infancy and childhood, and adult diabetes risk in five low- or middle-income country birth cohorts. *Diabetes Care* 35: 72–79.

Ochs, E., and L. Capps. 1996. Narrating the self. *Annual Review of Anthropology* 25: 19–43.

Ogden, C. L., M. D. Carroll, L. R. Curtin, M. A. McDowell, C. J. Tabak, and K. M. Flegal. 2006. Prevalence of overweight and obesity in the United States, 1999–2004. *Journal of the American Medical Association* 295(13): 1549–55.

Osborn, C., K. Patel, J. Liu, H. W. Trott, M. S. Buchowski, M. K. Hargreaves, W. J. Blot, S. S. Cohen, and D. G. Schlundt. 2010. Diabetes and co-morbid depression among racially diverse, low-income adults. *Annals of Behavioral Medicine* 41(3): 300–9.

Pabon-Nau, L., A. Cohen, J. B. Meigs, and R. W. Grant. 2010. Hypertension and diabetes prevalence among U.S. Hispanics by country of origin: The national health interview survey 2000–2005. *Journal of General Internal Medicine* 25(8): 847–52.

Pan, A., M. Lucas, Q. Sun, R. M. van Dam, O. H. Franco, J. E. Manson, W. C. Willett, A. Ascherio, and F. B. Hu. 2010. Bidirectional association between depression and type 2 diabetes mellitus in women. *Archives of Internal Medicine* 170(21): 1884–91.

Pennebaker, J. W. 1997. Writing about emotional experiences as therapeutic process. *Psychological Science* 8(3): 162–66.

Perez, A., H. Brown, and B. Restrepo. 2006. Association between tuberculosis and diabetes in the Mexican border and non-border regions of Texas. *American Journal of Tropical Medicine and Hygiene* 74: 604–11.

Peterson, K., J. Pavlovich, D. Goldstein, R. Little, J. England, and C. M. Petersen. 1998. What is hemoglobin A1c? An analysis of glycated hemoglobins by electrospray ionization mass spectrometry. *Clinical Chemistry* 44(9): 1951–58.

Petersen, K. F., and G. I. Shulman. 2002. Pathogenesis of skeletal muscle insulin resistance in type 2 diabetes mellitus. *American Journal of Cardiology* 90: 11g–18g.

Polletta, F. 2007. *It was Like a Fever: Storytelling in Protest and Politics*. Chicago: University of Chicago Press.

Polonsky, W. H., L. Fisher, J. Earles, R. J. Dudl, J. Lees, J. Mullan, and R. A. Jackson. 2005. Assessing psychosocial distress in diabetes. *Diabetes Care* 28: 626–31.

Ponce de Leon, A., L. Garcia Garcia, M. Garcia-Sancho, F. Gomez-Perez, and J. L. Valdespino-Gomez. 2004. Tuberculosis and diabetes in southern Mexico. *Diabetes Care* 27: 1584–90.

Popkin, B., S. Horton, S. Kim, A. Mahal, and J. Shuigao. 2009. Trends in diet, nutritional status, and diet-related noncommunicable diseases in China and India: The economic costs of the nutrition transition. *Nutrition Reviews* 59(12): 379–90.

Popkin, B., and J. Udry. 1998. Adolescent obesity increases significantly in second and third generation U.S. immigrants: The National Longitudinal Study of Adolescent Health. *Journal of Nutrition* 128(4): 701–6.

Porte Jr., D., D. G. Baskin, and M. W. Schwartz. 2002. Leptin and insulin action in the central nervous system. *Nutrition Reviews* 60(10, Pt. 2): s20–s29.

Portes, A., and R. L. Bach. 1985. *Latin Journey: Cuban and Mexican Immigrants in the United States*. Berkeley: University of California Press.

Poss, J., and M. A. Jezewski. 2002. The role and meaning of *susto* in Mexican Americans' explanatory model of type 2 diabetes. *Medical Anthropology Quarterly* 16(3): 360–77.

Pouwer, F., N. Kupper, and M. C. Adriaanse. 2010. Does emotional stress cause type 2 diabetes mellitus? A review from the European Depression in Diabetes EDID Research Consortium. *Discovery Medicine* 9(45): 112–18.

Radloff, L. S. 1977. The CES-D scale. *Applied Psychological Measurement* 1(3): 385–401.

Redfield, R., R. Linton, and M. Herkovits. 1936. Memorandum on the study of acculturation. *American Anthropologist* 38: 149–52.

Reissman, C. 1990. Strategic uses of narrative in the presentation of self and illness. *Social Science & Medicine* 30(11): 1195–1200.

Robinson, N., and J. Fuller. 1985. Role of life events and difficulties in the onset of diabetes mellitus. *Journal of Psychosomatic Research* 29: 583–91.

Rock, M. 2003. Sweet blood and social suffering: Rethinking cause-effect relationships in diabetes, distress and duress. *Medical Anthropology* 22: 131–74.

Rozin, P. 1996. Sociocultural influences on human food selection. In *Why We East What We Eat: The Psychology of Eating*, ed. E. D. Capaldi, 223–63. Washington, DC: American Psychological Association.

Rylko-Bauer, B., L. Whiteford, and P. Farmer. 2009. *Global Health in Times of Violence*. Santa Fe, NM: School for Advanced Research Press.

Sacks, D., D. Bruns, D. E. Goldstein, N. K. Maclaren, J. M. McDonald, and M. Parrott. 2011. Guidelines and recommendations for laboratory analysis in the diagnosis and management of diabetes mellitus. *Diabetes Care* 34: e61–e99.

Sampson, R., J. Morenoff, and T. Gannon-Rowley. 2002. Assessing neighborhood effects: Social processes and new directions in research. *Annual Review of Sociology* 28: 443–78.

Sapolsky, R. M. 2002. Chickens, eggs, and hippocampal atrophy. *Nature Neuroscience* 5(11): 1111–13.

Sapolsky, R. M. 2004. *Why Zebras Don't Get Ulcers.* 3rd edition. New York: Henry Holt and Company.

Scheper-Hughes, N. 1992. *Death without Weeping: The Violence of Everyday Life in Brazil.* Berkeley: University of California Press.

Scheper-Hughes, N., and P. Bourgois. 2004. *Violence in War and Peace: An Anthology.* Malden, MA: Blackwell Publishing.

Schoenberg, N., E. Drew, E. P. Stroller, and C. S. Kart. 2005. Situating stress: Lessons from lay discourses on diabetes. *Medical Anthropology Quarterly* 19(2): 171–93.

Schwab, T., J. Meyer, and R. Merrell. 1994. Measuring attitudes and health beliefs among Mexican Americans with diabetes. *The Diabetes Educator* 20(3): 221–27.

Sciolla, A., D. Glover, T. B. Loeb, M. Zhang, H. F. Myers, and G. E. Wyatt. 2011. Childhood sexual abuse severity and disclosure as predictors of depression among adult African-American and Latina women. *Journal of Nervous and Mental Disease* 7: 471–77.

Seeman, T. E., E. Crimmins, M.-H. Huang, B. Singer, A. Bucur, T. Gruenewald, L. F. Berkman, and D. B. Beuben. 2004. Cumulative biological risk and socio-economic differences in mortality: MacArthur studies of successful aging. *Social Science & Medicine* 58: 1985–97.

Seligman, R. 2005. From affliction to affirmation: Narrative transformation and the therapeutics of candomble mediumship. *Transcultural Psychiatry* 12(2): 272–94.

Shea, A., C. Walsh, H. MacMillan, and M. Steiner. 2004. Child maltreatment and HPA axis dysregulation: Relationship to major depressive disorder and post traumatic stress disorder in females. *Psychoneuroendocrinology* 30: 162–78.

Sherman, J., C. Carlson, J. F. Wilson, J. P. Okeson, and J. A. McCubbin. 2005. Posttraumatic stress disorder among patients with orofacial pain. *Journal of Orofacial Pain* 19: 309–17.

Simmons, J., and K. Koester. 2003. Commentary: Hidden injuries of research on social suffering among drug users. *Practicing Anthropology* 25(3): 53–57.

Simoons, F. J. 1994. Introduction. In *Eat Not This Flesh: Food Avoidances from Prehistory to the Present*, ed. F. J. Simoons, 3–12. Madison, WI: University of Wisconsin Press.

Singer, M. 1994. AIDS and the health crisis of the U.S. urban poor: The perspective of critical medical anthropology. *Social Science & Medicine* 39(7): 931–48.

Singer, M. 1996. A dose of drugs, a touch of violence, a case of AIDS: Conceptualizing the SAVA syndemic. *Free Inquiry in Creative Sociology* 24(2): 99–110.

Singer, M. 1997. Articulating personal experience and political economy in the AIDS epidemic: The case of Carlos Torres. In *The Political Economy of AIDS*, ed. M. Singer, 61–74. Amityville, NY: Baywood Publishing Company.

Singer, M. 2004a. Critical medical anthropology. In *Encyclopedia of Medical Anthropology*, eds. C. R. Ember and M. Ember, 23–30. New York: Springer.

Singer, M. 2004b. The social origins and expression of illness. *British Medical Bulletin* 69(1): 9–19.

Singer, M. 2009a. *Introduction to Syndemics: A Systems Approach to Public and Community Health*. San Francisco: Jossey-Bass.

Singer, M. 2009b. Desperate measures: A syndemic approach to the anthropology of health in a violent city. In *Global Health in Times of Violence*, eds. B. Rylko-Bauer, L. Whiteford, and P. Farmer, 137–56. Santa Fe, NM: School for Advanced Research Press.

Singer, M. 2011. Double jeopardy: Vulnerable children and the possible global lead poisoning/infectious disease syndemic. In *International Handbook on Global Health*, eds. R. Parker and M. Sommer, 154–61. London: Routledge.

Singer, M., F. Valentín, H. Baer, and Z. Jia. 1992. Why does Juan Garcia have a drinking problem? The perspective of critical medical anthropology. *Medical Anthropology* 14(1): 77–108.

Singer, M., and S. Clair. 2003. Syndemics and public health: Reconceptualizing disease in bio-social context. *Medical Anthropology Quarterly* 17(4): 423–41.

Singer, M., P. Erickson, L. Badiane, R. Diaz, D. Ortizb, T. Abraham, and A. M. Nicolaysen. 2006. Syndemics, sex and the city: Understanding sexually transmitted disease in social and cultural context. *Social Science & Medicine* 63(8): 2010–21.

Singer, M., and G. D. Hodge. 2010. *The War Machine and Global Health: A Critical Medical Anthropological Examination of the Human Costs of Armed Conflict and the International Violence Industry*. Lanham, MD: AltaMira Press.

Singer, M., A. Herring, J. Littleton, and M. Rock. 2011. Syndemics in public health. In *A Companion to Medical Anthropology*, eds. M. Singer and P. Erickson, 159–80. San Francisco: Wiley.

Soler, J., V. Perez-Sola, D. Puigdemont, J. Perez-Blanco, M. Figueres, and E. Alvarez. 1997. Validation study of the Center for Epidemiological Studies: Depression of a Spanish population of patients with affective disorders. *Actas Luso Exp Neurol Psychiatr Cienc Afines* 25(4): 243–49.

Strauss, A. L., and J. M. Corbin. 1990. *Basics of Qualitative Research: Grounded Theory Procedures and Techniques.* Newbury Park, CA: Sage.

Strosberg, A., and F. Pietri-Rouxel. 1996. Function and regulation of the β3-adrenoceptor. *Trends in Pharmacological Sciences* 17(10): 373–81.

Stunkard, A. J., and T. I. A. Sorensen. 1993. Obesity and socioeconomic status: A complex relation. *New England Journal of Medicine* 329: 1036–37.

Subramanian, S., I. Kawachi, and G. Davey Smith. 2007. Income inequality and the double burden of under- and overnutrition in India. *Journal of Epidemiology and Community Health* 61: 802–9.

Talbot, F., and A. Nouwen. 2000. A review of the relationship between depression and diabetes in adults: Is there a link? *Diabetes Care* 23: 1556–62.

Toobert, D. J., S. E. Hampson, and R. E. Glasgow. 2000. The summary of diabetes self-care activities measure. *Diabetes Care* 23: 943–50.

Trevathan, W. R., E. O. Smith, and J. J. McKenna, eds. 2008. *Evolutionary Medicine and Health: New Perspectives.* London: Oxford University Press.

Trief, P., P. Ouimette, M. Wade, P. Shanahan, and R. S. Weinstock. 2006. Post-traumatic stress disorder and diabetes: Co-morbidity and outcomes in a male veterans sample. *Journal of Behavioral Medicine* 29(5): 411–18.

Turner, B., K. Maes, J. Sweeney, and G. J. Armelagos. 2008. Human evolution, diet, and nutrition: When the body meets the buffet. In *Evolutionary Medicine and Health*, eds. W. R. Trevathan, E. O. Smith, and J. J. McKenna, 55–71. Oxford: Oxford University Press.

U.S. Census Bureau. 2010. Profile of General Population and Housing Characteristics: 2010 Demographic Profile Data for Chicago, Illinois. http://factfinder2.census.gov/.

Valdes, D. 2000. *Barrios Nortenos: St. Paul and Midwestern Mexican Communities in the Twentieth Century.* Austin: University of Texas Press.

Vega, W., A. Ang, M. A. Rodriguez, and G. K. Finch. 2011. Neighborhood protective effects on depression in Latinos. *American Journal of Community Psychology* 47(1–2): 114–26.

Walker, E., E. Newman, D. J. Dobie, P. Ciechanowski, and W. Katon. 2002. Validation of the PTSD checklist in an HMO sample of women. *General Hospital Psychiatry* 24: 375–80.

Watson, D., and L. A. Clark. 1984. Negative affectivity: The disposition to experience aversive emotional states. *Psychological Bulletin* 96(3): 465–90.

Weber, D. 1982. Anglo views of Mexican immigrants: Popular perceptions and neighborhood realities in Chicago, 1900–1940. PhD diss., Ohio State University.

Weiner, S., A. Schwartz, R. Yudkowsky, G. D. Schiff, F. M. Weaver, and J. Goldberg. 2007. Evaluating physician performance at individualizing care: A pilot study tracking contextual errors in medical decision making. *Medical Decision Making* 27: 726–34.

Weiner, S. J., A. Schwartz, F. Weaver, J. Goldberg, R. Yudkowsky, G. Sharma, A. Binns-Calvey, B. Preyss, M. M. Schapira, S. D. Persell, E. A. Jacobs, and R. I. Abrams. 2010. Contextual errors and failures in individualizing patient care. *Annals of Internal Medicine* 153(2): 69–75.

Weller, S., R. Baer, L. M. Pachter, R. T. Trotter, M. Glazer, J. E. G. Alba Garcia, and R. E. Klein. 1999. Latino beliefs about diabetes. *Diabetes Care* 22: 722–28.

Wilkinson, R., and K. Pickett. 2009. *The Spirit Level: Why Greater Equality Makes Societies Stronger.* New York: Bloomsbury Press.

Wilkinson, R. C. 1996. *Unhealthy Societies: The Afflictions of Inequality.* London: Routledge.

Wilkinson, R. G., and M. G. Marmot. 2003. *Social Determinants of Health: The Solid Facts.* Geneva, Switzerland: World Health Organization.

Willen, S. S. 2007. Introduction. In *Transnational Migration to Israel in Global Comparative Context*, ed. S. S. Willen, 1–27. Lanham: Lexington Books.

Willen, S. S., J. Mulligan, and H. Castañeda. 2011. Take a stand commentary: How can medical anthropologists contribute to contemporary conversations on "illegal" im/migration and health? *Medical Anthropology Quarterly* 25(3): 331–56.

World Health Organization. 2009. *Global Health Risks: Mortality and Burden of Disease Attributable to Selected Major Risks.* Geneva, Switzerland: World Health Organization.

Wynne, K., S. Stanley, B. McGowan, and S. Bloom. 2005. Appetite control. *Journal of Endocrinology* 184(2): 291–318.

Zimmet, P., K. G. M. M. Alberti, and J. Shaw. 2001. Global and societal implications of the diabetes epidemic. *Nature* 414: 782–87.

INDEX

abuse,
  emotional, 27, 59–62, 109
  interpersonal, 33–34, 36, 38–39,
    41, 43, 46–47, 50, 56–62, 77–79,
    89–91, 99–101, 107, 109, 119–20
  measurement of, 117
  physical, 12, 27, 36, 56–62, 78–79, 90,
    99, 118–19
  sexual, 11–13, 17, 24, 27–28, 36, 47,
    56–62, 69, 78–79, 88–90, 99–100,
    118–19
  substance, 22, 64, 66–67
  verbal, 59–62, 109
acculturation, 78, 82, 83–85, 99–100,
  106, 118
African Americans, 20, 112–13
age, 18, 20, 31, 41, 100
agency, 16, 89, 105
agricultural revolution, 94
AIDS/HIV, 22
alcoholism, 16, 22, 62, 64, 109
allostatic load, 98
American Indians, 115
anthropology,
  biocultural, 14,15
  critical medical, 14, 25
  medical, 14, 55
anthropometrics, 117
antidepressants, 50, 102, 104
anxiety, 43–46, 96
Anzaldúa, Gloria, 81

ataque de nervios, 54
atmospherics, 96

beliefs, cultural and folk,13, 54–56
biology of poverty, 113
biomedicine, 13, 21, 24–25, 105, 108,
  110–12
birthplace, 77–78, 99
blood pressure, 32, 96, 98, 103
body mass index (BMI), 32, 96, 117
Brazil,18

C–reactive protein (CRP), 103
carbohydrate metabolism, 95–96
Chicago, 23–26, 30–32, 34, 37–39, 42, 47, 66,
  68–69, 71, 73–76, 108–9, 112–13, 115
Chicagoacán, 30–31
childhood, 32–33, 38, 42–43, 45, 49,
  59–60, 77
  abuse, 11–12, 17, 23, 25, 27–28, 43,
    59–60, 77, 107
  memories, 11–12
children, 17, 31, 33, 39, 42, 65–69, 71,
  75–77, 108–9
China, 18
comorbidity, 14, 20–22
coraje (anger), 33, 54–56
corticotropin releasing hormone
  (CRH), 102
cortisol, 96, 102

culture, 26, 29, 55, 69, 108
cytokines, 102–3

depression, 11–14, 32, 38, 44–46, 107–8
    biology of, 95–96
    comorbidity with diabetes, 20–25, 44,
        54, 101–5, 107–8, 112–13
    measurement of, 30, 34, 64, 116
    predictors of, 68–69
    symptoms of, 28, 96–97, 99–101
    treatment of, 28, 110–12
developmental origins hypothesis,
    94–95, 119
diabetes, 11, 41
    biology of, 95–96
    cause/onset of, 21, 33, 44, 107
    comorbidity with depression, 20–25,
        44, 54, 101–5, 107–8, 112–13
    complications, 30, 32, 105, 108
    control, 46, 96–98, 117
    diagnosis, 35, 40, 43, 48–49
    disease of modernization, 17
    distress, 30, 43–44, 47, 49, 53–57,
        62–65, 78–79, 99, 101, 116–18
    duration of, 30, 116
    emergence of, 17–20, 73
    loss of someone as a result of, 69–70
    management of, 30, 40, 42, 49–50,
        65, 67, 72, 75, 104, 109
    severity of, 30, 116
    treatment of, 108–12
diet, 46, 67, 72–73, 82, 94–96, 103–4, 107,
    116. *See also* eating behaviors
discrimination, 15, 31, 47, 73–74, 108
distress, 12, 17, 21, 23–24, 46–49, 50, 54,
    62–64, 71, 82, 108, 119
    idioms of, 64–65
domestic violence. *See* violence
double burden of disease, 18, 113
drugs, 16, 22, 64–67, 75, 109

eating behaviors, 46, 67, 72–73, 82, 94–96,
    103–4, 107, 116. *See also* diet
economic development, 17–18, 94
education, 22, 31

embodiment, 24
emotion, negative, 35, 39, 41, 45, 48–50,
    55–65, 69–70, 78–79, 103–4,
    107–11, 113
empowerment, 24, 36
environment, 16, 24, 45, 55, 57, 73, 79
epidemic, 12, 17, 21–22, 26, 73, 78
epidemiology, social, 15, 24, 107
epigenetics, 95
epinephrine, 102
ethnicity, 79, 96
everyday violence. *See* violence
exercise. *See* physical activity

family, 27
    discord, 47, 57, 80, 109, 111
    income inequality, 19
    networks, 22, 30–32
    stress, 11, 16, 25, 34, 56–58, 65–67,
        78–79, 107
Farmer, Paul, 111
fat, 95–96, 103–4, 119
fibromyalgia, 62–64
fight or flight response, 102
folk beliefs and illnesses, 13, 54–56, 85–86
food deserts, 72–73
food insecurity, 72–73

gang, 22, 61, 66, 74–75, 80, 109
General Medicine Clinic, 28–31, 37, 42,
    50, 108
genetics, 94–95, 105
Ginicoefficient, 19, 115
glucose, 67, 95–96, 117
glucose transporters, 102
glycogen synthesis, 102
glycosylated hemoglobin, 116–18
grounded theory, 33–34, 51

health, 32
    behaviors, 105, 107
    mental, 14–15, 20, 28, 43, 49–50, 60,
        69, 96, 101, 109

outcomes, 34, 96, 101, 116
    physical, 14–15, 32, 49, 60, 62, 64,
        96, 101
health care, 29
    access to, 43, 48–50, 64, 105, 107–13
    diabetes and, 110
    psychological/psychiatric, 20, 48–50,
        108–9
hegemony, 15, 115
hemoglobin A1c, 117–18
HIV/AIDS, 22, 111
hypertension, 73, 103
hypothalamic-pituitary–adrenal (HPA)
    axis, 102

identity, 36, 65, 67
illegality, 108, 113
illness, 36, 46, 48
    constructions of, 36, 54–55
    narratives, 35, 36, 50, 62
immigration, 29–30, 32, 34, 46, 107–8,
    118–19
    stress, 56, 58, 61, 75–80, 113
    undocumented, 61, 74, 76–78,
        108, 115
    US–Mexican, 12, 23, 25–26
immodest claims of causality, 25, 55
India, 18
inequalities,
    gender, 15,
    health, 14, 113
    income, 19, 115
    political–economic, 17, 79, 107
    social, 79
    wealth, 15, 19, 113
inflammation, 102–3
influenza pandemic, 22
insecurity, economic, 80
institution, 42, 108, 111
    hegemony of, 15
    institutionalsupport, 24, 44, 46,
        49–50, 65, 75, 111
insulin, 95–96
    resistance, 13, 17–18, 95–96, 102–3
interleukin 6 (IL–6), 103

interpreter, 116
isolation. *See* social isolation

kidnap, 25, 42–43, 45, 61
Kim, Jim Yong, 111

Lancaster, Roger, 23
language, 29, 30, 50, 65, 73–74, 77–78,
    92, 99
Latino Health Paradox, 32, 82, 84, 89, 92
Latinos, 22, 29, 53
liberation theology, 15
life stories, 12–13, 25–28, 30, 33, 36, 38,
    46–47, 50
lifestyle, 15, 17–18, 94
Little Village, 31, 75, 91
Logan Square, 32, 75
loneliness, 56, 67–69, 117. *See also* social
    isolation
loss of a family member, 56, 69–71,
    99, 117

malnutrition, 22
Marxism, 15
medicine,
    adherence, 67, 103–4, 116
    prescription for, 110
memory, traumatic, 36, 47, 69, 77, 107
Mexican Chicago, 25, 30–32,
Mexico, 12, 18, 27, 30–32, 37, 61, 68–69,
    71, 75–76, 108–10, 117
Michoacán, 117
migration,
    chain, 30
    seasonal, 76
mind, 14, 49, 62, 113
modernization, 17, 18, 94
mortality, 21, 112
    all–cause, 32

narrative, 11–13, 24–26
    arc, 48
    illness, 35–36, 62

life history, 28–30, 33–34, 54, 56–57,
        108–10
    themes, 118
neoliberal economics, 13, 115
nervios (nerves), 54, 56
norepinephrine, 102
normalized violence. *See* violence

obesity, 17–18, 20, 32, 72, 80, 82, 94–98,
        103–5
oppression illness, 101

Partners in Health, 111
physical activity, 17–18,62, 65, 67, 82, 94,
        103–4, 107, 116
Pilsen, 31, 37, 75, 88
political–economic,
    environments, 16, 107–8
    inequality, 14–15, 17–18
    processes, 14, 16, 18, 36, 54–55, 105,
        113, 115
post–traumatic stress disorder, 28, 32, 34,
        64, 96–97
    measurement of, 117
poverty, 11–14, 22, 24–25, 31, 48, 62, 64,
        67, 71, 115
power, 16, 23, 47, 61, 89, 105, 109
psychiatry, 25, 28–29
psychotherapy, 30, 49–50
psychotropics, 104
public health, 54, 105
Puerto Ricans, 20, 22, 112–13

racism, 15–16, 53, 73–74, 87, 113
rape, 25, 38, 42–45, 61
resilience, 50

Sapolsky, Robert, 119–20
SAVA Syndemic, 22
self, 35–36, 42, 46, 48–49, 63, 107
Singer, Merrill, 12, 22, 93, 101, 105,
        107–8, 110, 115, 120
smoking, 103

social,
    detachment, 24, 68, 80
    inequality, 14
    integration, 26, 89, 92, 107
    isolation, 13, 23, 25, 34, 56, 58,
        67–69, 78–79, 88–92, 99–101,
        107, 112–13
    protection, 15, 46–47, 61, 108, 115
    networks, 13, 15, 17, 22, 26–27,
        30–31, 42, 61, 65, 74–75, 79, 100
    services, 28–29, 108, 112
    stress, 21, 25–26, 34, 54, 56–58, 64,
        77, 111
    suffering, 27–28, 64, 113
    support, 71, 77
social medicine, 113
South Chicago, 32, 75
Spanish, 23, 29, 31, 33, 49
stress, 17, 33
    cumulative effects of, 26, 73, 79,
        98–101
    diabetes, 11, 24, 56, 62–63, 99, 101
    family, 34, 56–58, 65–71,78–80,
        99, 107
    financial, 34, 56–58, 71–73,
        78–79, 99
    health, 14, 34, 56–58, 62–65,78,
        99, 101
    hormones, 96, 102–4
    immigration, 13, 23, 26, 34, 56–58,
        61, 75–80, 99, 113
    measurement of, 117
    neighborhood, 34, 56–58, 74–75, 78,
        91–92, 99
    nutritional, 94–95
    response, 102
    social, 21, 25–26, 34, 54, 56–58, 64,
        77, 111
    work, 34, 56–58, 73–74, 78, 80, 99
structural violence. *See* violence
sub–Saharan Africa, 18, 22
subjectivity, 42
subjugation, 15, 24, 61
suffering,
    psychological, 12, 27–29, 42, 50,
        63–64, 113

social, 18, 24–25, 27–29, 64, 113
strategic, 36
sugar, 62
susto (fright), 54–56, 109
symbolic violence. *See* violence
sympathetic nervous system, 102
syndemic, 21–25, 110–12
definition of, 12–13, 107–8
framework, 13, 21–22
interactions, 13, 22–23, 50, 107
model.*See* VIDDA Syndemic Model
SAVA, 22
theory, 21–25
VIDDA. *See* VIDDA Syndemic
synergistic interactions, 14, 21, 46, 113
synergy, 12

thrifty genotype hypothesis, 94
traumatic experience, 27, 33–34, 38–40,
42, 45–46, 49–50, 64, 76–77, 109
treatment, 36, 108, 110–12
tristeza (sadness), 56
tuberculosis, 18, 111, 113

undocumented, 47, 49, 61, 74, 76–70,
99, 113

unemployment, 42, 73
Uptown, 31, 75

values, cultural, 78
victimization, 17, 36, 50, 61
VIDDA Syndemic, 13–14, 23–26
application of, 112–13
construction of, 32–34, 36, 47, 50, 69,
74–75, 80, 107
definition of, 23–25
model, 105–6
theory, 13, 25, 36, 107
treatment for, 110–12
violence,
domestic, 36, 67, 115
everyday, 17
gender–based, 12, 17, 47, 56
invisible, 14
neighborhood, 25, 34, 74–75, 91–92
normalized, 17
structural, 13, 15, 17, 46–47, 55, 61,
73–75, 80, 111
symbolic, 13, 16–17, 47, 61, 107, 112

waist circumference, 96, 98, 117
wealth disparity, 13, 15
westernization, 94

ABOUT THE AUTHOR

Emily Mendenhall, PhD, MPH, a medical anthropologist, is a Research Fellow at the University of Witwatersrand in Johannesburg, South Africa, where she conducts research on women's health in Soweto. She has previously worked in Zambia, India, and the United States. Emily is also founder of a nonprofit committed to developing global health curricula for youth, and is the editor of two readers, *Global Health Narratives* (2009) and *Environmental Health Narratives* (2012) (www.GHN4C.org).